Nibblers Diet Plan

Ken Davies

Help4U Publishing

A catalogue record of this publication is available from the British Library

First Printed   2000
Revised Edition   2001

TRADEMARKS: Any product names mentioned within this publication may be trademarks or registered trademarks of their respective companies and are hereby acknowledged.

Although the author has researched the details presented in this book as thoroughly as possible, he assumes no responsibility for any errors, omissions or inaccuracies that may be contained therein. No liability can be accepted for any losses or expenses incurred as a result of relying on any information given therein.

ISBN 1842740261   Revised Edition

Internet: www.recipes4one.co.uk
Email: dietinfo@btconnect.com

Published by Help4U Publishing, Preston, UK.
http://www.help4u.net
Printed and bound by Antony Rowe Ltd, Eastbourne

Help4U Publishing

Acknowledgements

I would like to thank Helen and Ivy for their help in tasting the recipes for me.

Dedications

This book is dedicated to my wife Christine without whom this book would never of got started and for the support and understand she offered while I spent many hours writing it.

I would like to thank Helen and Ivy for their help in tasting the recipes for me.

Foreword

About You

"You just want Maximum results for the Minimum of effort."

You found losing weight to be problematical because most
diets plans work on three meals a day and you just like to
nibble all day.
Your are happy to exercise but it has to be little and often
spending hours exercising is just not your idea of fun.
You want tips on healthy snacks, advice on better eating habits

About the Diet Plan

This is a diet plan that is based on five small meals each day.
There are lots of instant snacks and recipes with many time
saving tips to get you in and out of the kitchen fast.
The diet plan offers you an easy exercises programme that does
not take you all day.
You are given advices on how to beat those hunger pains.

About the Author

The author is a registered Natural Health Practice Manager,
Weight Consultant, Nutritional Therapist, Vegetarian & Vegan
Nutrition, Herbalist, Women's Stress Practitioner, with
diplomas in Advanced Psychotherapy and Integrated
Therapeutic Counselling.

The author is also a member of the International Fitness
Association, an Aerobic & Fitness Instructor and a Step
Kickboxing Trainer and Sports Therapist.

Preface

This is a diet plan that is based on five small meals each day.
There are lots of instant snacks and recipes with many time
saving tips to get you in and out of the kitchen fast.
The diet plan offers you an easy exercises programme that does
not take you all day.
You are given advices on how to beat those hunger pains.

Contents

The Nibblers Diet Plan

Introduction

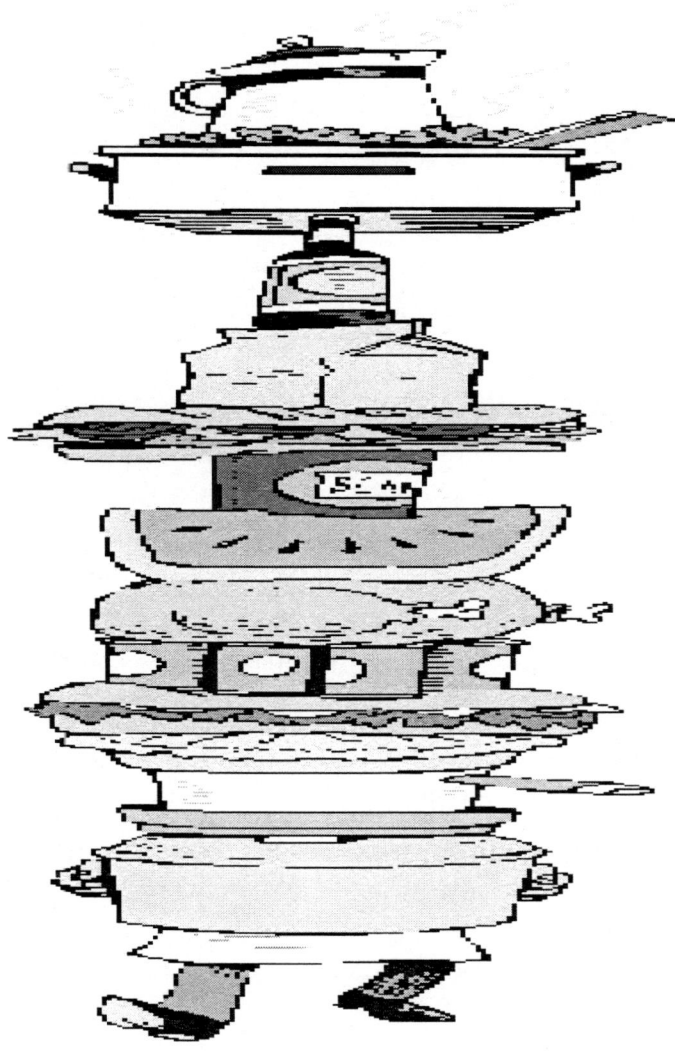

Introduction

As with any other diet plans if you have any doubts about your health before starting this diet plan please ask your doctor for advice. Also if you are pregnant or have an existing medical condition you should not follow the diet or exercise plan without first consulting your doctor. This diet plan is not recommended for children or people under sixteen years old.

- A warm welcome to **The Nibblers Diet Plan** this is one of a series of ten different style of diet plan books.

- Just what is different about this series of diet plan books?

- Well to start with all these diet plan books are published in a reader friendly format in a normal easy to read print version and a large print version.

- Each book offers you a diet plan to suit your personal lifestyle just choose the title that suits you the best.

- All the books in this series offer you a complete plan to help you succeed with your diet plan, fitness plan, and with building your self-confidence and self-assurance.

- The diet plans are not based on any crash diet; there is no counting of calories at all, no bizarre or special food combinations.

- I have just set out to help educate you to eat healthy and enjoy what you are eating.

- After your initial weight loss in the first two weeks, which is normally a larger amount because you will be losing water at this time, then it should fall to between 450g and 900g kg (1 to 2 lbs) per week.

If you lose any more you are risking losing muscle as well as fat, which is bad for your health and will slow down your weight loss in the long run.

- Just what could this diet plan mean to you, well this could be the end of that free size jogging suit you know the one you tell your self it has shrunk when you put weight on and you keep in the bottom draw for when nothing else fits.

- The end to panic when you are invited to a wedding, a party or when you are going on a holiday, about which of your clothes still fit you.

- The end to remorse and guilt after bingeing on your comfort foods and making those same resolutions each time something does not fit that you will this time lose weight.

- Increasingly today, we have become obsessed with our weight whether we consider our self to be over or underweight.

- With up to 65% of all women and 30% of all men in the UK have perceived that there is a problem with their weight and wish to do something about it.

- The UK population reportedly are spending over seven million pounds a week on diet food and diet drinks alone this provides a ready market.

- With peoples perception that they must be over weight or are not the right weight or look, this offers the industry a ready market.

- A lot of the population will buy anything if it is labelled to say low in fat, low in sugar, low in calories, this is played on by companies.

- The diet industries are moving to offer its products worldwide and are even happy to change their brand names to fit these markets.

- They are using the power of the label to say that the product is low in fat, low in sugar, low in calories, to play on the diet market.

They are also guilty of name changing to just give an old product a new name to improve product sales.

- Our fashion cultures has persuaded what it considers to be the desirable body shape with super models being given star status the populace are persuaded to think this is what they should look like.

- Peer pressures, the influence of family, friends, and partners. With the fact that everyone is or knows someone who is or has dieted it's hard not to get carried along to fit in.

- The television, movies, magazines, newspapers and the Internet showing or offering the slimming culture on a plate.

- As I cannot offer the keys to instant wealth there is no magic secret to losing weight and keeping it off.

- This is not one of them either as it does not ignore the inconvenient facts or avoid the unpleasantness that success in any endeavour requires coming to terms with the true nature of the task at hand and the problems causing it.

- How can I lose weight when I am told by the anti diet faction that over 98% of all diets simply do not work and in fact cause you to gain more weight in the long run.

- I am also told how the fashion industry and the media have in part created the eating disorders such as anorexia nervosa and bulimia and are being taken to task over this by the government.

- So any suggestion that I should try to control my world seem pointless even dangerous to my health.

- I have after all tried lots of other slimming, weight loss diets and these never worked at all or did work only for a short time but I soon put all the weight back on and some extra as well.

- I expect you would say that in your experience 100% of diets just do not work at all.

- Despite this there is unquestionable clinical evidence that weight loss diets do work.

The simple truth is, take in fewer calories than your body needs to maintain your current weight and you will unquestionably lose weight.

- A very simply way to workout your approximate average daily calories intake is to just add a nought to your weight in pounds thus if you weight 210 pounds you need to take in 2100 calories to maintain this weight.

- So by taking in fewer calories than your body needs or by undertaking some exercises you will lose weight.

- This is surely great news for the majority of basically healthy people who would like to not only to lose weight but also keep it off permanently because all they need to do is to find away of reducing their calorie intake and increasing the calories they burn.

- But you say "I only have to look at a cream cake and I put on weight" this may be equally applied to any food the fact is that you are under estimating the total amount of calories in your present diet and on eating extra to your daily needs the body just stores the extra.

- The facts are that being overweight is not only be harmful to your health but, is cost you money, and may be why you have such low self-esteem.

- A study from Cambridge University found that the more overweight a person was the greater they underestimated their daily intake, with an average overweight person eating 40% more than they need to maintain a stable weight level.

How To Stop Smoking and Lose Weight

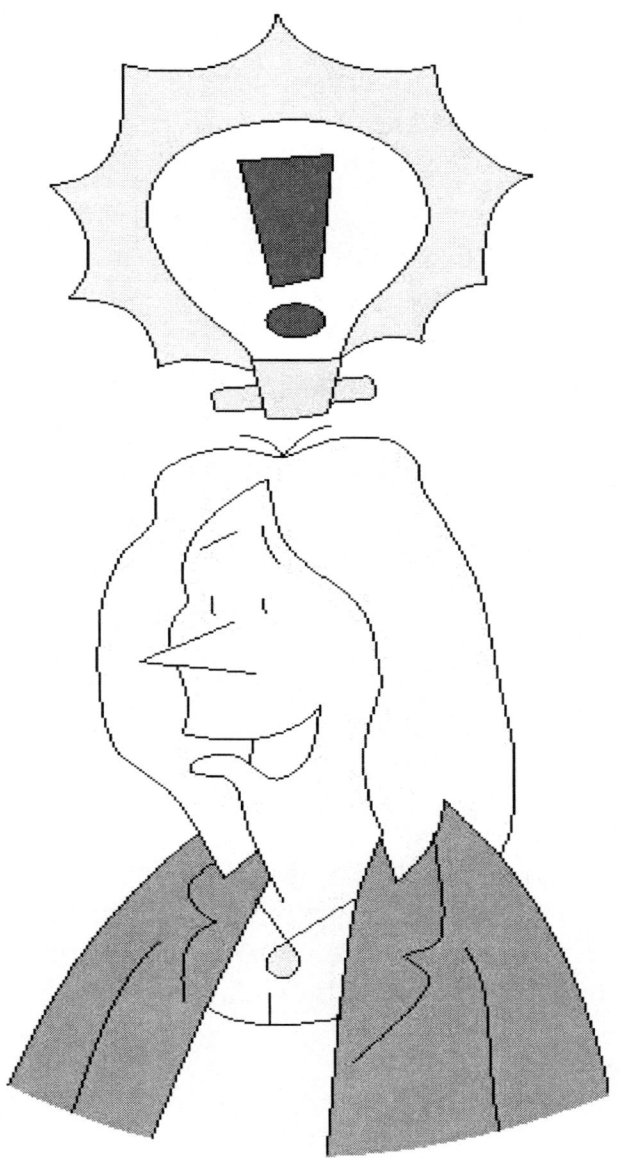

How to Stop Smoking and Lose Weight

I am offering you a way to help you take control of not only your eating habits but also many other problems you may have. So why not plan to stop smoking at the same time and start a new life today.

- I understand that your particular concern may be the possibility of weight gain if you stop smoking.

- Yes it is true that weight gain is common immediately after stopping smoking it is on average about only 6-8 lbs, but this is the weight gain made without any attempts at dieting or exercise.

- This in its self presents only a minor health risk when compared to the risk of continued smoking.

- The reasons for weight gain are not fully understood at this time, it may be partly explained by the fact that smoking increases the body's metabolic rate that is the rate at which calories are burned up.

- In addition it is thought that nicotine may act as an appetite suppressant so that when smokers quit an increase in appetite leads to an increase in calorie intake.

- This may also explain why smokers tend to weigh less than non-smokers.

- Do smokers wish to give up; well it has been found that more than 71% of all adult smokers would like to give up? It has been establish that the more a person smokes the less faith that he or she has that they can stop.

The most important element of the stopping smoking seems to be the smoker's own decision to quit.

Time since quitting	Beneficial health changes that take place
Within 20 minutes	The body begins a series of changes that continues for years. Blood pressure and pulse rate return to normal. Body temperature of hands and feet increases to normal.
Within 8 hours	Nicotine and carbon monoxide levels in blood reduce by half, oxygen level increases to normal.
Within 24 hours	Carbon monoxide will be eliminated from the body. Lungs start to clear out mucus and other smoking debris. Chances of a heart attack decreases
Within 48 hours	There is no nicotine left in the body. Ability to taste and smell is greatly enhanced improved. Nerve endings start re-growing.
Within 72 hours	Breathing becomes easier. Bronchial tubes begin to relax and energy levels increase.
Within 2 - 12 weeks	Circulation improves. Walking becomes easier. Lung function increases up to 30%.
Within 3 - 9 months	Coughing, sinus congestion, fatigue, shortness of breath decreases. Cilia re-grow in your lungs, increasing your ability to handle mucus to clean the lungs, and reduce infection. Body's overall energy increases
Within 1 years	Risk of a heart attack falls to about half that of a smoker.
Within 5 years	Lung cancer death rate for the average smoker (20 per day) decreases by almost half. Stroke risk is reduced to that of a non-smoker 5-15 years after stopping. Risk of cancer of the mouth, throat and esophagus is half that of a smoker's
Within 10 years	Lung cancer death rate similar to that of a non-smoker. Risk of cancer of the mouth, throat and esophagus, bladder, kidney and pancreas decreases.

Prepare to Stop Smoking

Lets look at what you must do first, you will need to prepare mentally, but remember about three million of Britain's smokers try to quit each year and there are more than 12 million people in Britain have become successful ex-smokers.

- Nevertheless, it can be tough and you will need lots of willpower to break the hold of nicotine, a powerful and addictive drug.

- First you will need to draw up a plan of action, considering what help and methods are available to you.

- Then make a date and stick to it, this should be the start of your diet plan.

- You will need to keep busy to help take your mind off cigarettes.

- Make your home a no smoking area; throw away all your ashtrays, lighters, and unopened cigarette packets, just keep one cigarette.

- Lets take a moment to look at what else giving up smoking can do for you.

- You will benefit by having better all round health by stopping smoking.

- The risk of a heart attack drops to that of a non-smoker after three years of quitting.

- The risk of cancer drops with every year of not smoking.

- You can live longer and stay well.

- You will after all be setting a good example for your children or other peoples children, I am sure you do not want to be seen as smoking role model.

You should now have more money to spend on other things as an average smoking 20 a day can cost about £1,522 per year.

Cigarettes	Years of smoking				
Per day	1	5	10	20	50
5	£381	£1,903	£3,805	£7,610	£19,026
10	£761	£3,805	£7,610	£15,221	£38,051
20	£1,522	£7,610	£15,221	£30,441	£76,102
40	£3,044	£15,221	£30,441	£60,882	£152,205

- You will now have a better chance of having a healthy baby

- All of your food and drink will now taste better.

- Your skin and complexion will improve and there should be no early wrinkles. You will have a fresher smelling breath, hair and clothes and an end to that cigarette smells around the house.

- What if you do not stop well one in two long-term smokers will die early and lose about 16 years of life.

- Treat yourself, this is important if you can, use the money you are saving by not smoking to buy something special big or small that you usually would not have.

- Be careful what you eat follow your chosen diet and excise plan.

- Involve your friends or family if you live with someone else that smokes, it will be much easier to quit if you do it together.

- A common mistake is not to take the effort to quit smoking seriously enough, putting your whole commitment behind it will help you have the right frame of mind to face the challenge and succeed.

- Whilst it is good to smoke fewer cigarettes rather than more, cutting down is less likely to work than simply stopping outright.

Unfortunately, even if you do manage to cut down, the numbers tend to creep back up again.

- So once you have planned ahead and chosen your date it is better to stop outright.

- With 75% of all ex-smokers said that the method that helped them to quit was their own willpower.

- Its not easy but possible as to date more than 12 million people in Britain have now become successful ex-smokers.

This Is Time For Your Very Last Cigarette Ever

Today is the day you will stop smoking, now this is time for your very last cigarette every, you may light up but as you smoke it please think just how much this habit has cost in money and your health.

- You now just need to follow this diet plan you will need to make sure that you drink plenty of fluids, water is cheap or any low calories drink will do.

- By undertaking the exercise plan that accompanies the diet plan of your choosing this will help you not only to relax but can boost your morale.

- You need to think positively, withdrawal can be unpleasant but it is a sign your body is recovering from the effects of tobacco.

- Irritability, urges to smoke and poor concentration are common do not worry; they usually disappear after a couple of weeks.

- Try to change your routine it helps to try and avoid the shop where you usually bought your cigarettes.

- Also you should try to avoid the pub or the break room at work if there are lots of smokers around you.

- Try doing something totally different take a new sport or just start going for a walk.

- There are no possible excuses please do not use a crisis or even good news to be an excuse for just one you will soon want the next and the next.

- Please just take one day at a time each single day without a cigarette is good news for you and your health, your family and your pocket.

Boosting Your Self Esteem

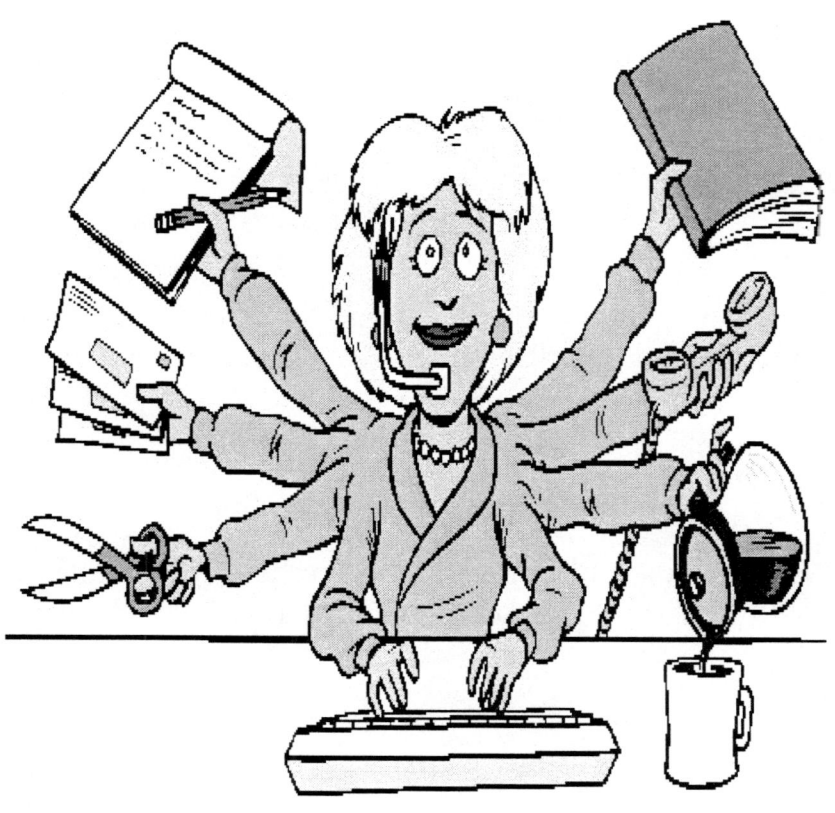

Boosting Your Self Esteem

Are you self critical and pre-judgmental, find yourself running around trying to please everyone and in the end pleasing no one at all, not even yourself.

- Do you at times feel that the world and every one in it are against you?

- You find that you do not bounce back like you once did, when you take yet another one of lives hard knocks.

- This all sounds very familiar the chances are you have a very low self-esteem, and this may be part of why you are over weight.

- You need to beware how damaging low self-esteem can be and understand the difference between self-esteem and confidence.

- Do you put on a brave face or show of confidence generally most of us do, but this is all just superficial.

- Where as your confidence can be synthetic you cannot pretend to feel good about yourself with a low-esteem.

- A high level of self-esteem acts like a shield or a shock absorber.

- If at a party or when you are out someone passes a tactless remark, it is your confidence acts as your shield or shock absorber it takes the blow, but having a low level of self-esteem and you take yet another one of life's hard knocks.

- Getting through life without the support of self esteem will be very challenging to say the least, you will find that you need to use artificial props to fill gaps and offer the appearance of confidence you present to the world.

To compensate some just keep themselves extremely busy, others will just drink excessively, or take drugs while a lot turn to eating or in fact overeating.

- It is the use of this prop food and overeating that confirms you have a poor opinion of yourself.

- I hope to help you to help yourself overcome this overeating as this can only make your self-esteem lower still.

- To help you combat your overeating and get this diet plan to work for you we need you to try to increase your level of self-esteem so you will not be dependent on food to fill the gaps in your life.

- But if you have low self-esteem how is this going to be possible, I imagine you will usually tend to bottle up your all your negative emotions instead of facing up to them.

- The first and most important step is for you to be recognise your negative and positive feelings and how to deal with them face on.

- Are you trying to silence your emotions by visiting the refrigerator? Could it be this simply YES! Could be.

- You ought be dealing with any of your problems head on by what ever means, this could be by just having a good cry right away or by containing it until a more appropriate time to release it.

- This may be hard for you especially if you come from a background were any show of environment or strong feelings were frowned on.

You can learn a lot from stormy types who throw cushions around or cry at that soppy, gushy, slushy, sentimental film or book.

- On being able to learn to show emotions you will feel strong inside and this will help you overcome your over-eating problem.

- Look for the real you is a magnificent and unique being with enormous potential and capacity for experiencing love of yourself and extending love to others.

- As your self-esteem grows, the real you emerges you will begin to take more risks and not be afraid of failure; you are not as concerned with getting approval of others; so your relationships are much more rewarding; you pursue activities that bring you joy and satisfaction; and you will make a positive contribution to the world.

- Most importantly of all, high self-esteem brings you peace of mind when you're alone; you truly appreciate the person you are with yourself.

- First and foremost stop putting yourself down you cannot develop a high self-esteem if you constantly think negative thoughts about yourself and your abilities.

- Whether speaking about your appearances, your career, your relationships, your financial situation, or any other aspects of your life, avoid putting yourself down.

- You must stop comparing yourself to other people if we all look we will always find someone who has more than you and some who have less.

- All compliments received should be accepted with just "thank you." If you replied with," Oh, it was nothing." you are rejecting this worthy compliment.

Also by playing down a compliment the message you give yourself is that you are not worthy of praise "not true is it".

- Use positive statements to enhance your self-esteem.

- Write out a statement such as these on the back of a business card or small index card carry the card with you. "I am truly a valuable and lovable person that deserve the best in life" or "I am truly going to succeed and stop smoking for good" or "I will truly follow this diet plan and succeed".

- Repeat the statement several times during the day, especially at night before going to bed and after getting up in the morning.

- Whenever you say the affirmation, allow yourself to experience positive feelings about your statement.

- Most people will dwell on their inadequacies and then wonder why their life is not working out.

- Make a list of your positive qualities, are you honest, helpful, artistic, creative, thoughtful, unselfish write down at least 21 of your positive qualities.

- It is important to review this list often and start focusing on your positive qualities and you will stand a much better chance of achieving them.

- Be true to yourself and live your own life not the life others have decided is best for you.

- You can never gain your own self-respect and feel good about yourself if you aren't leading the life you want to lead.

If you're making decisions based on getting approval from friends and relatives, you are not being true to yourself and your self-esteem will be lowered.

- If you only watch negative television programs or read newspaper reports of murders and business rip offs; you will grow cynical and pessimistic.

- Similarly, if you read books or listen to programs, that are positive in nature, you will take on these characteristics. Associate with positive, supportive people.

- Being surround constantly by negative people who put your ideas down and your self-esteem is lowered. On the other hand, when you are accepted and encouraged, you feel better about yourself in the best possible environment to raise your self-esteem.

- Start giving more of yourself to those around your when you do things for others, you are making a positive contribution and you begin to feel more valuable, which in turn, lifts your spirits and raises your own self-esteem.

- You must take positive action, as you cannot develop high self-esteem if you sit on the sidelines and back away from challenges.

- When you take action regardless of the ensuing result you will feel better about yourself.

- When you fail to move forward because of fear and anxiety, you'll be frustrated and unhappy and you will undoubtedly deal a damaging blow to your self-esteem.

- Try to get involved in work and activities you love it is hard to feel good about yourself if your days are spent in work you despise.

Self-esteem will flourishes when you are engaged in work and activities that you enjoy and make you feel valuable.

- Even if you cannot explore alternative career options at the present time, you can still devote leisure time to hobbies and activities, which you find stimulating and enjoyable.

How To Beat Stress

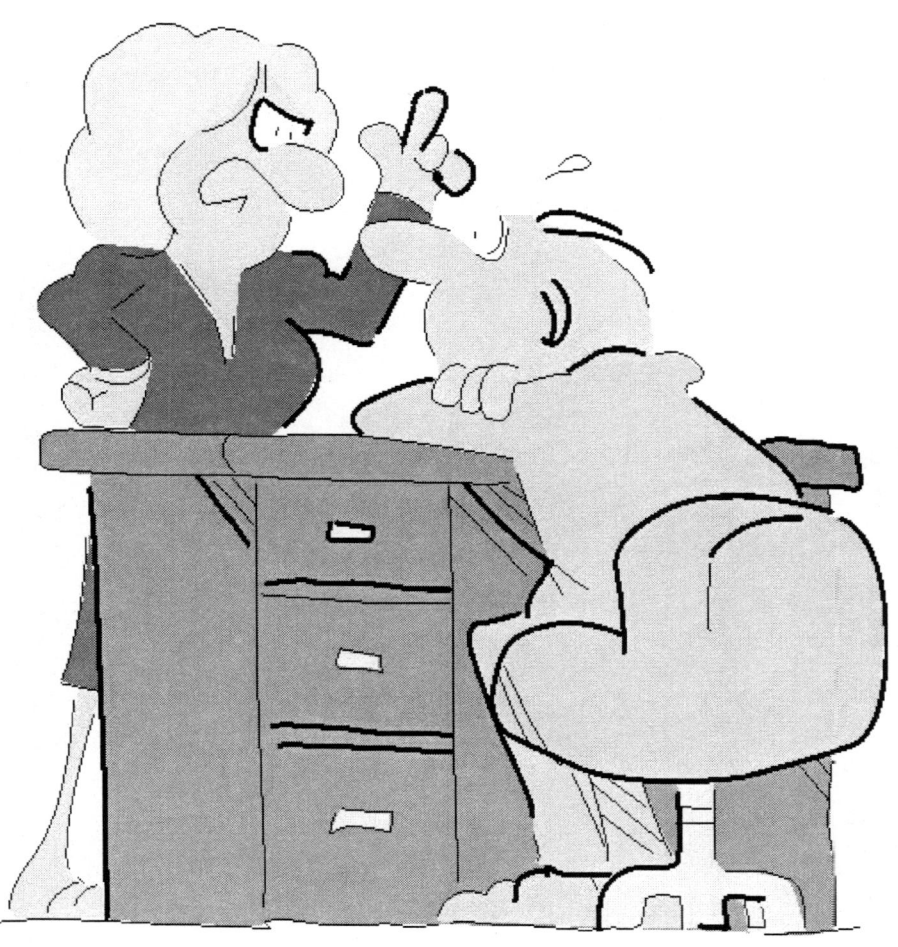

How To Beat Stress

If you are going to beat stress you must first understand just what it is and why it is important to us.

- You cannot have failed to notice that life is stressful and that stress now a days seems to come at us from all directions.

- As long as you are alive stress cannot be avoided only reduced. Life without some stress would be boring we certain need an amount of stress to creates motivation and challenge.

- What is every day stress like then just recall the last time you were perhaps driving a car when someone suddenly pulled out in front of you.

- Or you were confronted with an immediate threat, and your body instantly goes into action this is called "fight or flight" this is the physiological, psychological response to a threat.

- This is left over from our distant past when this very often was the key to life or death.

- So just what is going on before you can think or act your body as already done lots of things.

- What do you remember your body doing as it went into a heightened state of physiological arousal to help you deal with this threat?

- You may have noticed an increase in muscle tension. In a threatening situation you may have to defend yourself, so there is a generalized increase in muscle tension.

- Your reflexes will be faster when your muscles are slightly tense. It is like the stance of a runner at the start of a race.

- Your body is set to go and increased muscle tension prepares you for the needed action.

- Your increase in muscle tension prepares you to act but as your muscles tense you will need more oxygen.

Your heart rate goes up to more quickly to pump the oxygen carrying red blood cells to the muscles.

- You may notice the pounding in your chest and your heart rate increases; there is also a corresponding increase in your blood pressure.

- Your breathing pattern changes and respiration becomes more rapid and shallow as more oxygen is brought into your lungs, and then picked up by the blood cells, which take it to your muscles.

- As all of this activity is going on it is not a good time to be leisurely digesting food as your gastrointestinal system comes to a screeching halt as the blood supply is diverted away from the belly to the large muscles of the body that are preparing for action.

- You may notice the "butterflies in the tummy " sensation these physical changes are the ones we are most aware of when confronted with a threat, especially, if the threat is dangerous.

Many other processes are going on but are out of awareness.

- For example, the pupils of the eyes dilate so that you can see well.

- Chemical reactions occur so that you blood will clot faster, and you will not bleed to death if cut defending yourself.

- The blood vessels in the extremities constrict so that not as much blood flows, and you would bleed less if cut.

- In addition to all these physical changes you may notice emotional changes as well.

- Most often people feel either angry or afraid.

- Well, with this as a reminder of what you body does, when you are threatened, lets' ask, why do we in fact look for stressfully things to undertake.

- Think about that visit to an amusement park to ride the roller coaster, or other rides then you have been seeking stress.

During these activities your body will be showing all the physiological indicators of stress.

- However, if we ask what you are doing, you will probably reply that you are, "having fun." Since you have voluntarily entered the situation you found it exciting, fun, and a challenge and you feel in control.

- If someone was making you do these things against your will then you might be terrified.

- What types of stress are there, well stress comes in two-category positive stress, which is called eustress, and negative stress, which is distress.

- Positive stress is what turns you on, and distress is what wears you out.

- Positive stress involves such changes as getting married, having a baby, or accepting a promotion that requires you to relocate.

- With positive stress as we adapt and adjust we feel competent, challenged, and satisfied with our ability to cope.

- But negative stress comes from changes or changes that cannot be avoided, change itself is not the problem.

- Change has always been with us what has happened is that "the type of change" has changed, it has become more rapid events will not slow down again.

- We are living in what we will soon look back on as, "the good old days" when things were slow.

- As the rate of change increases so does the level of distress.

- Most modern stress comes from the social framework in which we live and the psychological and emotional reactions to them.

- It has been estimated that only about 10% or less of modern stress comes from actual physical threat to life.

- The other 90% comes from the perception of life events.

Such sources of stress are financial worries, job conflict, aging parents, and children having trouble in school, health problems and crime.

- These problems do not easily go away and are hard to fight against.
- You cannot run away from them and often take them wherever you go.

Just what are there symptoms:

- Tightening of your muscles.
- Raising your heart rate and blood pressure.
- Creating a rapid breathing pattern.
- Shutting down digestion.
- Bringing about emotional distress such as anger, anxiety frustration.

And producing physical symptoms such as.

- Asthma.
- Back pain.
- Coronary heart disease.
- Diabetes.
- Hypertension (high blood pressure).
- Indigestion.
- Irritable bowel syndrome.
- Migraine.
- PMS.
- Rheumatoid arthritis.
- Skin disorders.
- Stomach ulcers.

Stress also depresses the function of the immune system and so lowers our resistance to common ailments such as colds and flu.

- Stress also has been implicated in the development of certain cancers.

- And of course it aggravates all manner of mental and emotional disorders, as well.

- Learn to laugh, as it is one of the healthiest antidotes to stress.

- Get rid of your anger, as it is the single most damaging stress-related personality trait that precedes a heart attack.

- You can learn to take control of the events in your life that are causing you stress so that you have less stress.

- Try to establish routines as people who have high stress level in their lives tend to live surrounded by mental and physical chaos.

- Be assertive you must stand up for your decisions, and express your feelings, and be able to accept, and give compliments.

- Be decisive as indecision prevents you from taking action and causes a loss of a sense of control and thus intensifies your stress.

- With effort some on your part you should be able to pinpoint specific settings, relationships, and people that are stressful.

- You must get adequate sleep as lack of adequate sleep can make you moody, angry and more vulnerable to illness.

- You should be able to avoid some situations or at least not intensify them reduce, control, or eliminate some stressors in an intimate relationship.

- No matter what happens to us we always have to think about it before we react.

- Writing down your feelings in a diary may help relieve emotional stress this is especially helpful if you trouble talking about your problems.

- If you live in a noisy house of flat and are continually disturbed by your neighbours, you could try to move someplace quiet.

Adopting a realistic attitude to life and its events can reduce stress just do not make things worse than they are.

- By developing a positive attitude much of your stress can be reduced.

- Encourage yourself think in positive terms about your self-will higher your self-esteem and lower your stress levels.

- Accept family members for the way they are they are not about to change just because you want them to.

- Stay healthy and stress resistant by taking time out for meals, eating at regular times.

- If you are stressed out and need a break from anxiety, try foods low in fat and protein and high in complex carbohydrates for a calming effect.

- You can use exercise to work away your tension and fortify yourself against the negative physical effects of stress, try an aerobic activity or just take a walk; swim.

- Relax by breathing deeply.

Understanding Craving and Bingeing

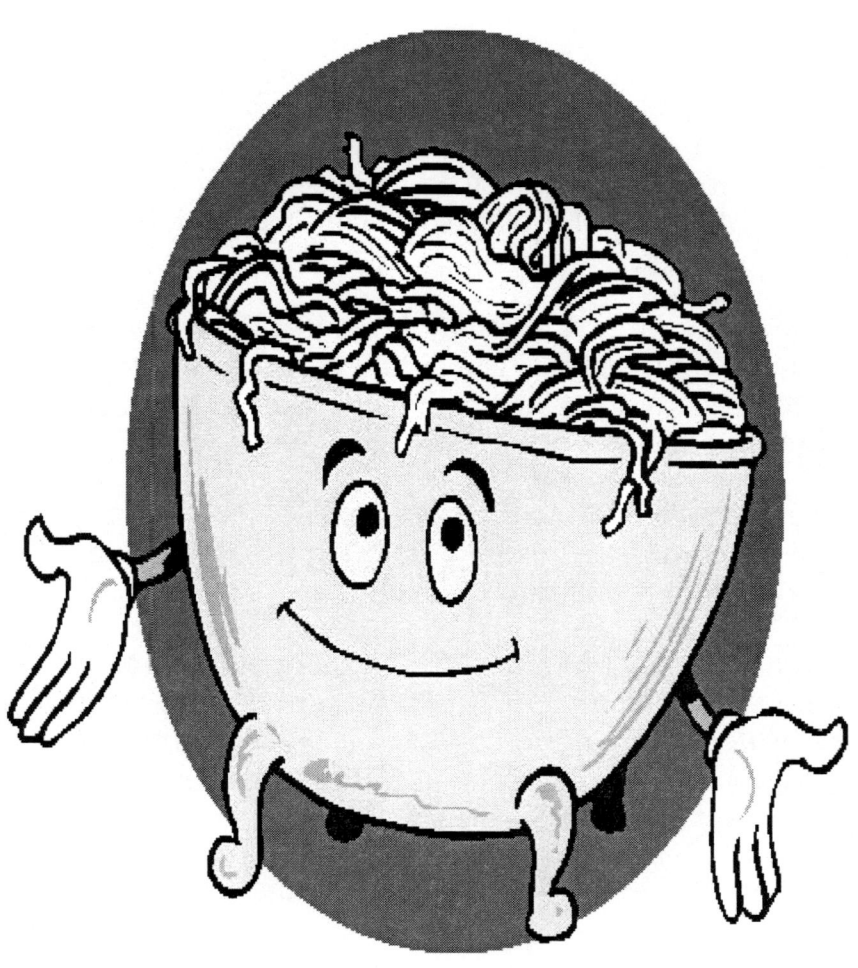

Understanding Craving and Bingeing

You will in all probability start on this diet plan as you have probably done on many others having told yourself this time it will work, you will loose some weight then out of the blue bang your favourite food starts calling you.

- So why do we have cravings and end up bingeing why do we have this problem and when and where did it all start.

- Why does this happen well the association between food and comfort begin in our infancies when as a baby we cried, we were given a bottle or feed, so we quickly learn to associate food as a relief of stress and frustration not just as a relief of hunger.

- This association was continually reinforced throughout our childhood for example, as a crying child we were given such things as chocolate, ice cream, biscuits or milk to comforted you.

- So not surprisingly these particularly foods that we were given for comfort, as a child are often the very same comfort foods we turn to as an adults.

- As you will now see there is in fact a built in associated with food and happy emotion from birthdays to weddings as well as negative emotion ones such as being stressed, frustrated or with funerals and wakes as these are all celebrated with food.

- You would of found that traditional diets set you up for this because it is deprivation that ultimately results in powerful cravings.

- Nearly everyone who has dieted can tell his or her own version of the same sad story.

Most people cannot successfully achieve significant and lasting weight loss by the daily ritual of self-denial called dieting, because physiological urges beyond their control eventually overpower any willpower.

- So after failing to stick to a diet or, even more frustrating, after successfully losing weight, you have helplessly watched the pounds pile back on as your eating when out of control.

- Why should you believe that this diet will work, this is not a diet but a diet plan for your lifestyle, you select which diet plan to follow the one that suites your life style best.

- So what can you do to beat craving and bingeing?

- You may have had a stressful day at work or in the home, someone may have said or done something to hurt your feelings, you may be feeling lonely, lost, isolated, fed up or just bored.

- Whatever the reason, it's important that you have a plan to prevent the binge from taking place.

- A good idea would be to make up a list of things to do to help prevent you from bingeing and keep this list handy so that it can be accessed whenever the urge to binge arises.

- Here is my own list of a few alternatives to bingeing that you may find helpful and may want to include on your own list.

- Sit down and try to understand the reasons why you want to binge and write in your diary how you are feeling at this moment.

- Make a list of foods you are planning to binge on, seal them in an envelope and throw it out or burn it.

- Call a friend or logon to a chat room on the Internet.

Go for a walk or try to leave the surroundings that are tempting you to binge or just visit a friend.

- Try to get your mind on something else read a magazine or a book please but not food or cookbooks do a crossword, some crafts or jigsaw puzzle.
- Take a long bath to relax or try some deep breathing exercises.
- Put on some of your favourite music, shut yourself in your room and dance and sing to it with your eyes closed.
- If you love music and have extra time, learn to play a few songs with an instrument and practice when you feel like bingeing.
- Pamper yourself polish your nails, get your hair done or get a massage or take up yoga or a stress relieving class.
- Write a long letter or e-mail to a friend or family friend.
- If you have a quote the gives you strength when you read it, recite it to yourself when you are feeling down.
- Draw or colour a picture of something powerful or trying playing with your dog or petting your cat if you have a pet.
- If you enjoying gardening, get involved in planting a garden, or rearrange or redecorate a room.
- Learn to relax and slow down by using exercise, yoga or meditation.
- Take deep breaths, close your eyes, and picture yourself in a field or at a beach. Turn on quiet music; any method of relaxation helps.

Begin an enjoyable task or project immediately after eating a meal.

- Carry food to work rather than buying it there.
- Pack healthy, satisfying food.

Is Your Anger Making You Fat

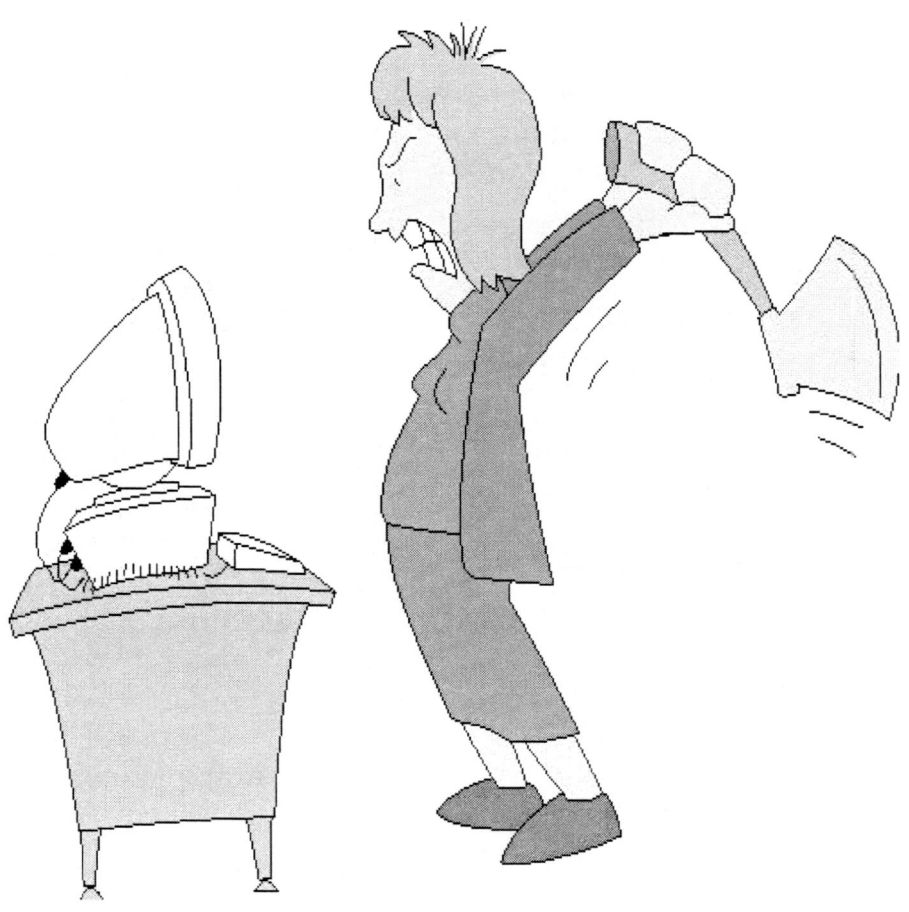

Is Your Anger Making You Fat

Could it be possible that it is your anger that is making you overeat? Just think about it do you never get angry, annoyed, irritated, heated, cross, furious, or gnashing your teeth or are you just unable to express your anger.

- You do still feel it but because you are suppressing your anger you need to look to a way to lessen your frustration and you are turning to food.

- Do you find yourself with half eaten foods in front of you not remembering having eaten them while furious about some injustice at home or at work.

- You could be using food to diffuse your anger or just block it out.

- While there are many types of anger we are only concerned with hidden or suppressed anger and as such, it as been named passive aggressiveness.

- Such persons engaging in passive aggressiveness may be unresponsive, argumentative, and overly nice, play dumb, arrive late, exaggerate the faults of others, and engage in nasty gossip that is hurtful.

- Also passive aggressiveness can morph itself into silence, lack of communication, tiredness, anxiety, high blood pressure, heart disease, depression, guilt, self defeating behaviour such as resorting to drinking, food or drugs, submissiveness, crying, or in its extreme form, paranoid schizophrenia.

- You may feel that there is nothing you can do to change the situation and just accept it. Here are some approaches that may be found to be helpful.

- Try to reduce your frustrations find the source of your frustration, whether they are people, subjects or situations and attempt to reduce or eliminate your exposure.

Make time for yourself each day and no one else

- Reduce violent stimuli in your life choosing to avoid violent movies; violent and aggressive friends are part of this approach.

- Be very selective with your friends so that they do not goad you into anger and rage.

- Eliminate drugs and alcohol as stimulants of anger.

- Reveal yourself and understand others announce you may be having a bad day to others.

- Attempt to indicate to others that they are having a bad day and offer to listen or let them vent.

- Stop hostile fantasies and dwelling on issues or people that aggravate you think tranquil, think calm.

- Do not escalate the violence by aggressive action on your part as this may cause an equally aggressive response, which starts a vicious cycle.

- Suppress or convert your violent reaction, count to ten, take a deep breath, think calmly about a "a ribbon of sand between the angry sea and the placid bay"; "the quiet waters of a lagoon"; "a lake of tranquil blue water reflecting a tranquil blue sky".

- Think of the source of the aggravation and whether a violent reaction will accomplish any purpose other than remorse, which is not a goal.

- Stop using temper to get your way while successful in the short term, using anger to win points is a losing strategy in the long run.

- Consider meditation and other mild exercise to help you relax.

Strategies For Dealing With PMS

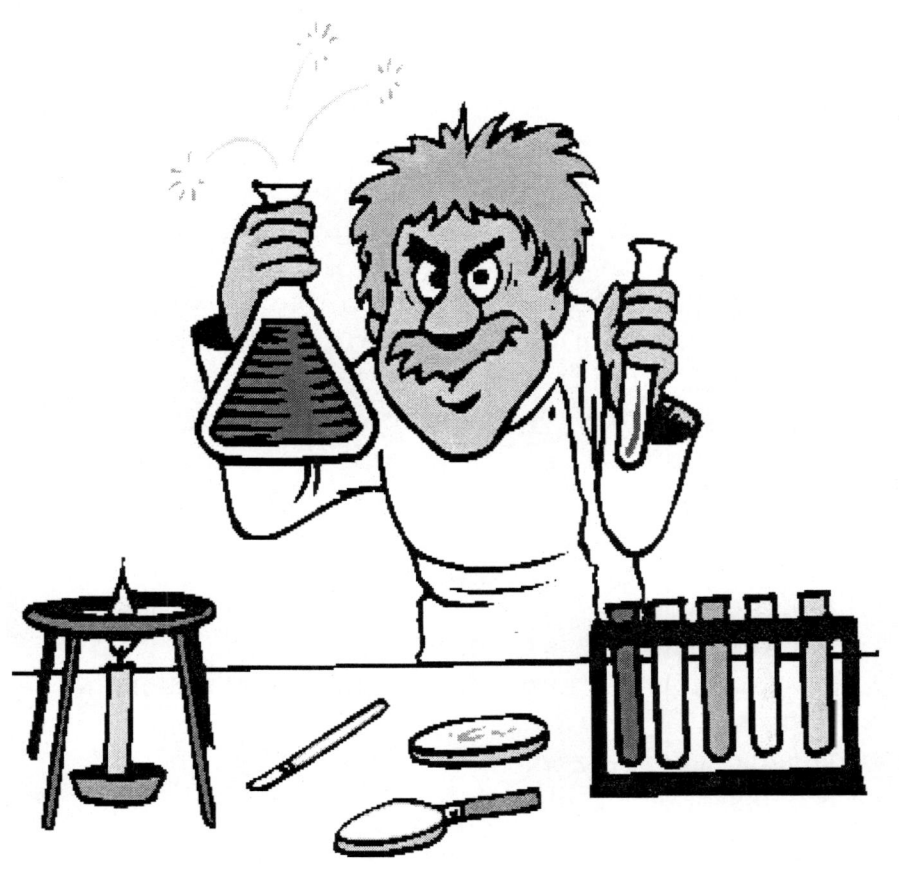

Strategies For Dealing With PMS

Having knowledge about PMS ought help you understand, accept and manage this condition. Try to encourage your partner, family and friends to understand by telling them how you are feeling and by sharing your knowledge. Seek support from other women and from the people you live with.

It has been suggested by medical research that over 40% of all women of child bearing age could suffer seriously from PMS, pre menstrual syndrome that will cause them real distress. It is also understood that many others could suffer adversely affected to a lesser extent for the few days before a period with symptoms such as feeling weepy, tired and irritable. It is at this time when many women will turn to comfort eating or have craving for high sugar foods and chocolate. So could this be why you have problem in the past sticking to a diet.

Some women experience only a few symptoms, while others may have many of them. The discomfort felt as a result of PMS symptoms ranges from mild to so severe that it might interfere with everyday activities. What are the symptoms of Pre-Menstrual Syndromes in fact has a series of symptoms that appear before the menstruation these may include:

- Depression
- Irritability
- A propensity towards outbursts of anger
- Distention tenderness and pain in the abdomen and breasts
- Headache and dizziness
- Restlessness and insomnia
- Water retention
- Diarrhoea
- Increase in appetite
- Cravings mainly for sweet or salt foods
- Weight gain
- Tiredness
- Low blood sugar

What is the cause of PMS there are several theories about why PMS occurs with some researchers believe that PMS is triggered by fluctuations of the sex hormones during the menstrual cycle. They believe a drop in progesterone levels or the increase in oestrogen levels during the latter half of the menstrual cycle may be responsible. Another theory holds that vitamin deficiencies may be the culprit a deficiency of vitamin B6, for example, may be responsible for the depression and mood fluctuations of PMS. Yet another theory links PMS with sudden changes in the body's levels of certain morphine-like substances as it is suspected that changes in the female hormones produce fluctuations in the levels of these opiates that influence appetite and moods.

How is PMS treated I am sorry to say there is no single cure for PMS nevertheless many women, have found that making changes to their lifestyle can help to control the symptoms these include:

- Try to just take life easy, plan ahead so you can avoid late nights.
- A diet low in salt and refined sugar and high in breads, cereals, fruit and vegetables should help.
- Reducing your intake of caffeine in such things as coffee, tea, cola and chocolate.
- By eating small meals more often, may help reduce the symptoms of insomnia, anxiety and mood swings.
- Try to reduce smoking and alcohol consumption.
- Wear loose clothing if you suffer from abdominal bloating and a well supporting bra for breast tenderness.
- Try a gentle massage or heat as it can relieve abdominal discomfort or back pain.
- Many women have found that acupuncture and naturopathy helps relieve PMS.
- Taking regular exercise, be in control of PMS; do not let it control your life.

Relaxing Your Body and Calming Your Mind

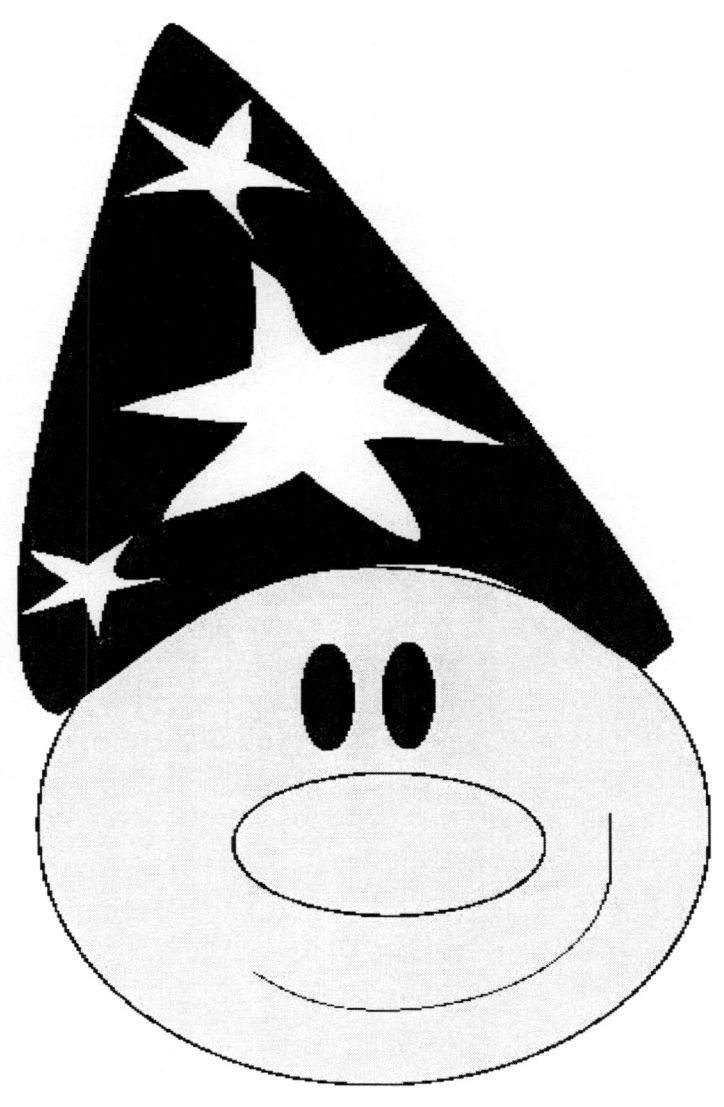

Relaxing Your Body and Calming Your Mind

Generally people today are so caught up with what is occurrence around them such as the latest news on the TV that e-mail message appearing on your computer screen that you have forget to pay attention to what's happening in your own mind, body, and heart. Here are some ways to relax that have been found to work.

- When at work try and find a place where you can have some peace and quiet sit quietly close your eyes if this helps and think of some that you enjoy such as music, a movie, a person, or somewhere you travel too or would like to, a few minutes can relax you profoundly.

- Try just calling someone to chat it needs to be with someone who will be happy to hear from you and who will not dump their stress on you, this can be a parent, a spouse or friend tell them you are calling to relax and take your mind off your day. Try telling jokes, talk about anything that is fun, relaxing, or interesting your call should last for at least ten minutes.

- At home turn on your answering machine or turn off your telephones ringer and take timeout, find the quietest and most comfortable area and sit or lay down close your eyes and listen to relaxing music and think only of things you love to do, see, or experience. Take pleasure in the moments and the images allow your muscles to relax and your eyes to rest.

- Learning how to calm the mind and body through meditation or self-relaxation. Once learned, it can be used virtually anywhere and at any time.

- Avoid anything with caffeine or nicotine or alcohol in it. Eat a healthy snack as stress depletes us of vitamins, minerals, blood sugar and calories. A healthy snack like a piece of fruit, a small chocolate bar, a glass of fruit juice or skimmed milk can revive us. If these are eaten or drunk slowly in a quiet atmosphere they can recharge our emotional and physical batteries.

Try just taking a 10-minute spin in your car on as quiet and uncontested a road as possible. If the weather is good, roll down the window and breathe in the fresh air.

- Keep your eyes on the road of course listen to a music tape you like if you feel like it, sing along with the music, look at the landscape, the clouds in the sky.

- You should come home happy and relaxed.

- After a stressful day at work take a warm long shower and use aromatic shower gel, or take a long warm bath add herbal bath salts and let the water relax your muscles listen to some relaxing music light a scented candle if you wish and just let the stress dissolve into the water and be washed.

- When using your home or works computer take at least 10 minutes out to play a quiet, non violent game, you are not worry about winning or even finishing the game, just have fun.

- Try exercising taking a walk, riding an exercise bike, take up yoga, or other aerobic activity will help rid your body of a lot of stress you will find that you are more relaxed and more alert.

The Nibblers Diet Plan

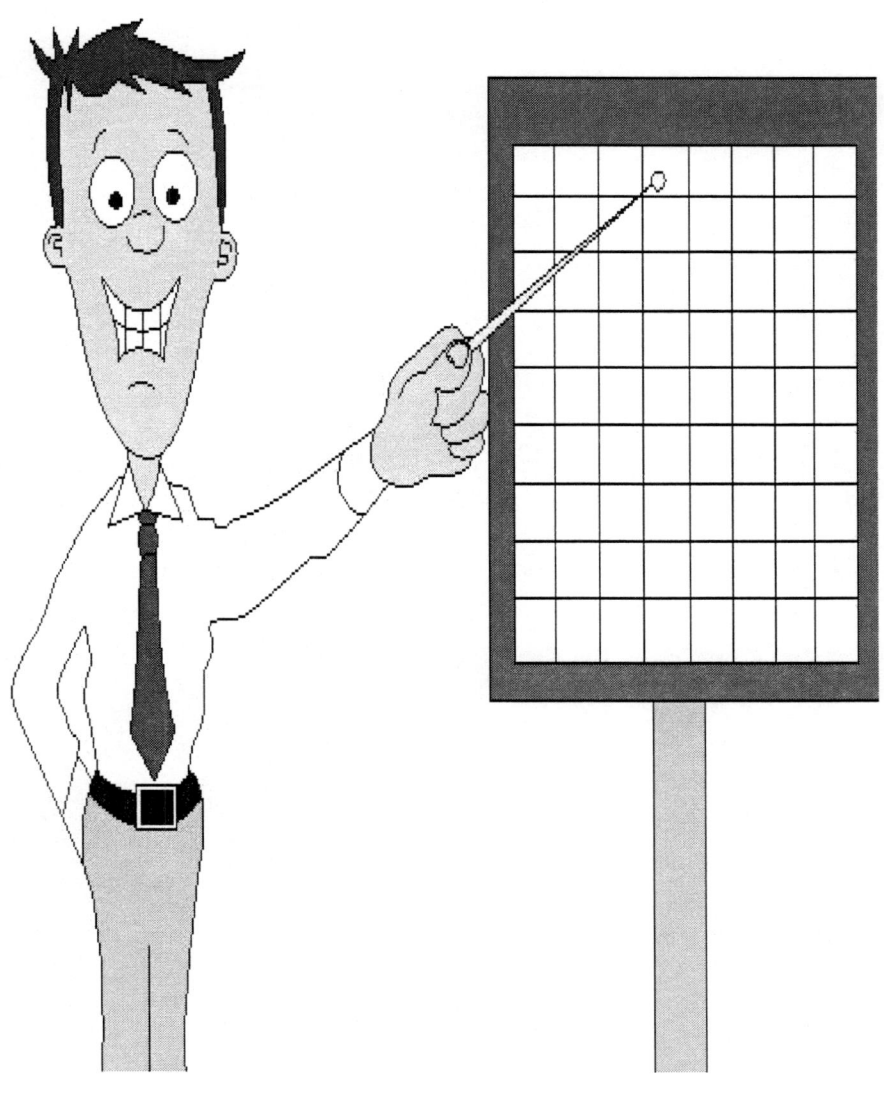

Weight Chart

Women		Height		Men	
Weight Range				Max Weight	
Metric	Imperial	Imperial	Metric	Imperial	Metric
45.5 – 50.0	07.02 – 07.12	4' 10"	1.47	08.08	54.3
47.2 – 51.8	07.06 – 08.02	4' 11"	1.50	08.12	56.2
48.6 – 53.6	07.09 – 08.06	5' 0"	1.52	09.02	58.1
50.5 – 55.5	07.13 – 08.10	5' 1"	1.55	09.06	60.0
52.3 – 57.3	08.03 – 09.00	5' 2"	1.57	09.10	61.8
53.6 – 59.1	08.06 – 09.04	5' 3"	1.60	10.01	64.1
55.5 – 60.9	08.10 – 09.08	5' 4"	1.63	10.05	65.9
57.3 – 62.7	09.00 – 09.12	5' 5"	1.65	10.10	68.2
59.1 – 64.5	09.04 – 10.02	5' 6"	1.68	11.01	70.5
60.9 – 66.4	09.08 – 10.06	5' 7"	1.70	11.05	72.3
62.7 – 68.6	09.12 – 10.11	5' 8"	1.73	11.10	74.5
64.5 – 70.5	10.02 – 11.01	5' 9"	1.75	12.01	76.3
66.4 – 72.7	10.06 – 11.06	5' 10"	1.78	12.06	79.1
68.2 – 75.0	10.10 – 11.11	5' 11"	1.80	12.11	81.4
70.0 – 76.8	11.00 – 12.01	6' 0"	1.83	13.02	83.6
72.2 – 79.1	11.05 – 12.06	6' 1"	1.85	13.07	85.9
74.2 – 81.3	11.10 – 12.11	6' 2"	1.88	13.12	88.2
76.2 – 83.5	12.00 – 13.02	6' 3"	1.90	14.04	90.9
78.3 – 85.7	12.05 – 13.07	6' 4"	1.93	14.09	93.2

The Nibblers Diet Plan

Here's what to do

You found losing weight to be problematical because most diets plans work on three meals a day and you just like to nibble all day.

Your are happy to exercise but it has to be little and often spending hours exercising is just not your idea of fun.

You want tips on healthy snacks, advice on better eating habits This is a diet plan that is based on five small meals each day.

There are lots of instant snacks and recipes with many time saving tips to get you in and out of the kitchen fast.

The diet plan offers you an easy exercises programme that does not take you all day.

You are given advices on how to beat those hunger pains..

YOU DO NOT HAVE TO COUNT CALORIES ON ANY OF MY DIET PLANS THAT IS DONE FOR YOU.

Try to choose different meals each day to get your full daily nutrimental requirements.

It does not mater which order you eat the meals just simply fit them around your daily routine.

Please do try to spread them over the whole day and just eat them at one time.

If you do not wish to eat five meals a day them you can combine two of them together

After checking you weight on our Weight Chart if you are one stone of less over weight then each day just choose five meals from the meal list 1 to 5.
One meal from list 1.
One meal from list 2.
One meal from list 3.
One meal from list 4.
One meal from list 5.
Plus your daily allowanc.

After checking you weight if you are one to three stone over weight then each day just choose.
One meal from list 1.
One meal from list 2.
One meal from list 3.
One meal from list 4.
One meal from list 5.
One extra meal from list 1.
Plus your daily allowance.

After checking you weight if you are more then three stone over weight then each day just choose.
One meal from list 1.
One meal from list 2.
One meal from list 3.
One meal from list 4.
One meal from list 5.
One extra meal from list 1 and 2.
Plus your daily allowance.

Daily Allowance

You are allowed up to the following each day

- ½ pint of skimmed milk; this can be UHT long life skimmed milk, this is for you to use in with any cereal, or in your tea, or coffee
- 1 small pot of diet yoghurt
- 2 oz of a low fat spread
- 2 pieces of average fruit
- As many cups of tea or coffee with milk from your daily allowance
- You may have a hot bed time drink if you wish but please use a low calorie one
- As many low calorie soft drinks as you wish
- As much water tap or bottled as you can drink

Before Pictures

Please select a current photograph and stick the chosen photograph here then take another after and stick it along side the other.

Date ....

Weight ....

Chest/Bust ....

Waist ....

Hips ....

After Picture

Date ....

Weight ....

Chest/Bust ....

Waist ....

Hips ....

Your Progress Chart

	Weight Now	Weight Loss	Your Measurements Bust/Chest	Waist	Hips	Exercise Done
Week 1						
Week 2						
Week 3						
Week 4						
Week 5						
Week 6						
Week 7						
Week 8						
Week 9						
Week 10						
Week 11						
Week 12						
Week 13						
Week 14						
Week 15						
Week 16						
Week 17						
Week 18						
Week 19						
Week 20						
Week 21						
Week 22						
Week 23						
Week 24						
Week 25						
Week 26						

Your Progress Chart

	Weight	Weight	Your Measurements			
	Now	Loss	Bust/Chest	Waist	Hips	Exercise Done
Week 27						
Week 28						
Week 29						
Week 30						
Week 31						
Week 32						
Week 33						
Week 34						
Week 35						
Week 36						
Week 37						
Week 38						
Week 39						
Week 40						
Week 41						
Week 42						
Week 43						
Week 44						
Week 45						
Week 46						
Week 47						
Week 48						
Week 49						
Week 50						
Week 51						
Week 52						

BMI Chart

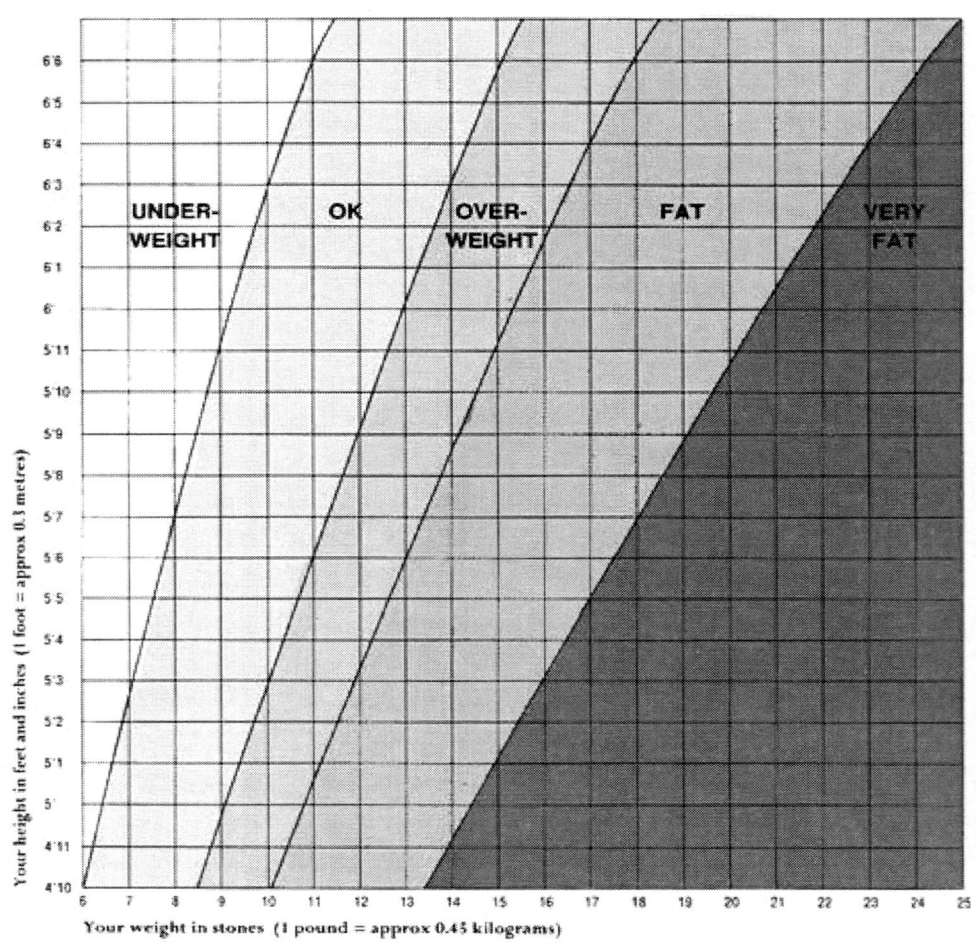

Your height in feet and inches (1 foot = approx 0.3 metres)

Your weight in stones (1 pound = approx 0.45 kilograms)

☐ **Underweight** Are you eating enough?

☐ **OK** This is the desirable weight range for health.

▢ **Overweight** Not likely to have much effect on your health but don't get any fatter!

▨ **Fat** Your health could suffer if you don't lose weight.

■ **Very fat** This is severe and treatment is urgently required.

MEAL LIST 1

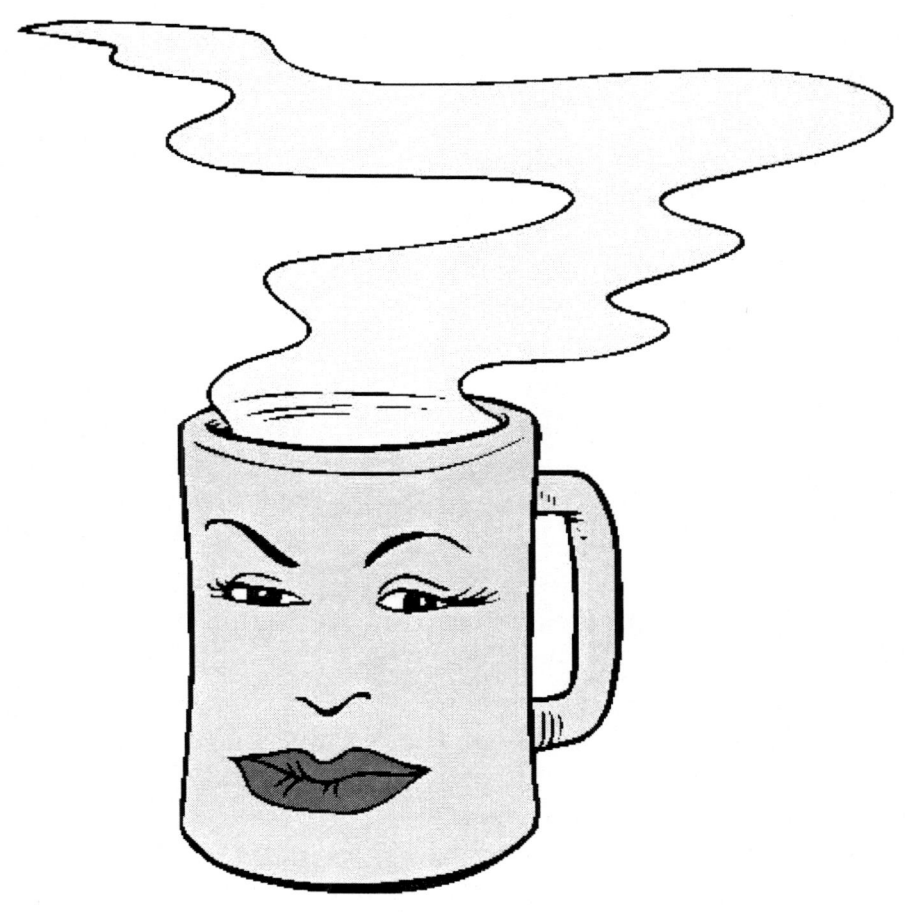

MEAL LIST 1

One box of Choco Corn Flakes taken from Kellogg's Variety Pack with milk taken from the daily allowance.

One box of Frosties taken from Kellogg's Variety Pack with milk taken from the daily allowance.

One box of Corn Flakes taken from Kellogg's Variety Pack with milk taken from the daily allowance.

One sachet of Bran or Apple & Cinnamon Quaker Oatso Simple made with milk taken from the daily allowance.

One sachet of Honey Bran Quaker Oatso Simple made with milk taken from the daily allowance.

One sachet of Original Quaker Oatso Simple made with milk taken from the daily allowance.

One box of Corn Pops taken from Kellogg's Variety Pack with milk taken from the daily allowance.

One box of Choco Krispies taken from Kellogg's Variety Pack with milk taken from the daily allowance.

One box of Nesquik from Nestle Pic-a-Pac with milk taken from the daily allowance plus .

One box of Honey Nut Cheerios from Nestle Pic-a-Pac with milk taken from the daily allowance.

One box of Shreddies from Nestle Pic-a-Pac with milk taken from the daily allowance.

MEAL LIST 1

One box of Honey Nut Shredded Wheat from Nestle Pic-a-Pac with milk taken from the daily allowance.

One box of Rice Krispies taken from Kellogg's Variety Pack with milk taken from the daily allowance.

One box of Honey Loops taken from Kellogg's Variety Pack with milk taken from the daily allowance.

One sachet of Golden Syrup Quaker Oatso Simple made with milk taken from the daily allowance.

----

1 whole fresh pink grapefruit and a boiled egg with a slice of wholemeal bread spread with low fat spread.

----

1 whole fresh pink grapefruit and a slice of wholemeal bread spread with honey or jam.

----

1 slice of wholemeal bread toasted and spread with low fat spread top with a cooked turkey rasher.

2oz / 50g of any muesli with milk taken from the daily allowance.

2oz of Kellogg's Fruit and Fibre with milk taken from the daily allowance.

----

1 slice of wholemeal bread toasted and spread with low fat spread top with 1 cooked turkey rasher, 1 grilled tomato.

MEAL LIST 2

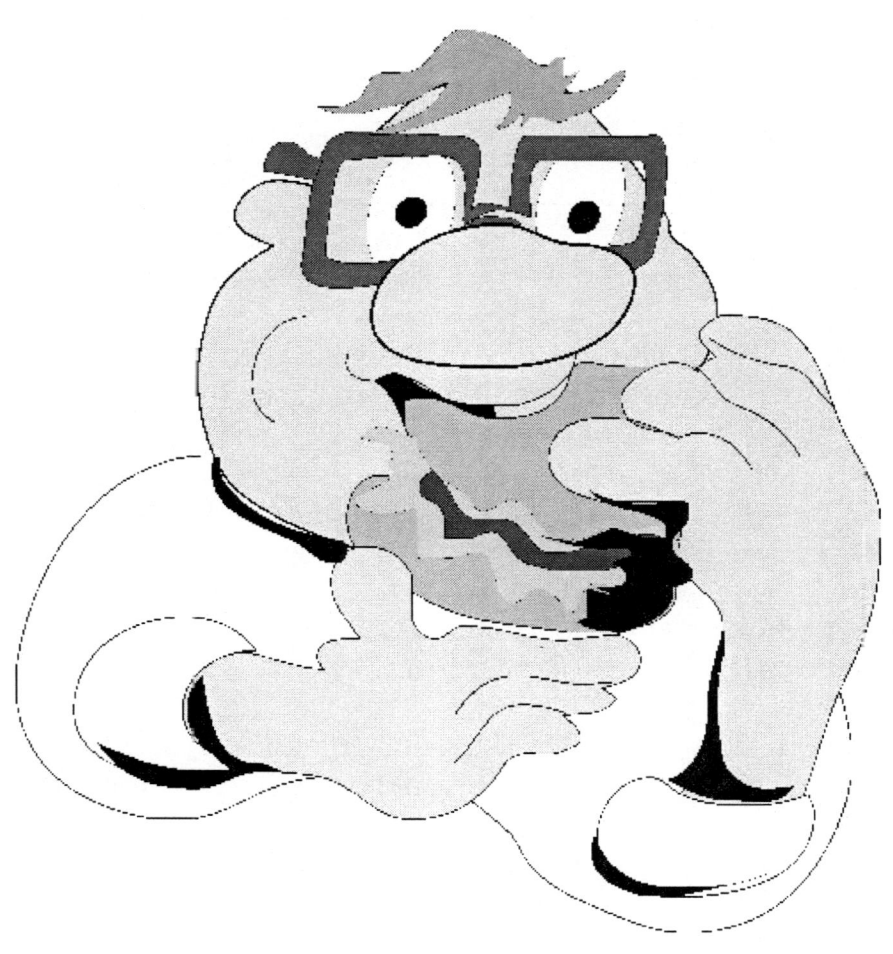

MEAL LIST 2

1 slice of wholemeal bread toasted and spread with low fat spread top with 1oz of lean ham plus 1 sliced tomatoes.

----

1 slices of wholemeal bread toasted and spread with low fat spread top with a cooked turkey rasher 7oz tin of mushrooms.

----

1 slice of wholemeal bread toasted and spread with low fat spread top with one poached egg.

----

2 slice of wholemeal bread toasted with 2 teaspoons of marmalade or jam.

2oz of Kellogg's All-Bran with milk taken from the daily allowance.

----

1 slice of wholemeal bread toasted and spread with low fat spread top with a 7oz / 200g can of cooked tomatoes and a cooked turkey rasher.

2oz of Kellogg's Special K with milk taken from the daily allowance.

----

1 slice of wholemeal bread toasted and spread with low fat spread and half a fresh pink grapefruit.

----

1 slice of wholemeal bread toasted and spread with low fat spread top with 2 cooked turkey rashers and 2 grilled tomatoes.

----

1 slice of wholemeal bread toasted and spread with low fat spread top with a 4oz of heated tin tomatoes, a poached.

MEAL LIST 2

11oz can of Breakfast Compote in Apple Juice.

----

2 cooked turkey rashers 1 slices of wholemeal bread toasted and spread with low fat spread.

2oz of Kellogg's Sultan Bran with milk taken from the daily allowance.

2oz of Grape Nuts with milk taken from the daily allowance.

Half a fresh pink grapefruit and a 5oz diet yoghurt.

7oz of smoked haddock cooked in milk taken from the daily allowance.

----

1 slice of wholemeal bread toasted and spread with low fat spread top with a 7oz / 200g can of heated tin baked.

----

1 Kellogg's Nutri-Grain Apple Bar.

----

1 Kellogg's Nutri-Grain Blueberry Bar.

----

1 Kellogg's Nutri-Grain Cherry Bar.

----

1 Kellogg's Nutri-Grain Strawberry Bar.

----

1 Muller Light Blueberry Yoghurt.

----

1 Muller Light Banana Yoghurt.

MEAL LIST 2

1 Muller Light Strawberry Yoghurt.

----

1 Muller Light Apple Yoghurt.

----

1 Muller Light Vanilla Yoghurt.

----

1 Muller Light Cherry Yoghurt.

----

1 Muller Breakfast Bio Pear Yoghurt.

----

1 Muller Breakfast Bio Maracuya Yoghurt.

----

1 Tesco Healthy Eating Bio Morello Cherry Yoghurt.

----

1 Tesco Healthy Eating Bio Nectarine and Orange Yoghurt.

----

1 Tesco Healthy Eating Bio Raspberry Yoghurt.

----

1 Tesco Healthy Eating Bio Strawberry Yoghurt.

----

1 Tesco Healthy Eating Bio Toffee V.

----

1 Tesco Healthy Eating Bio Tropical Yoghurt.

----

1 Tesco Healthy Eating Bio Vanilla Yoghurt.

----

1 Tesco Healthy Eating Custard Style Gooseberry Yoghurt.

----

1 Tesco Healthy Eating Custard Style Plum Yoghurt.

----

1 Tesco Healthy Eating Custard Style Rhubarb Yoghurt.

----

1 Tesco Healthy Eating Custard Style Strawberry Yoghurt.

MEAL LIST 3

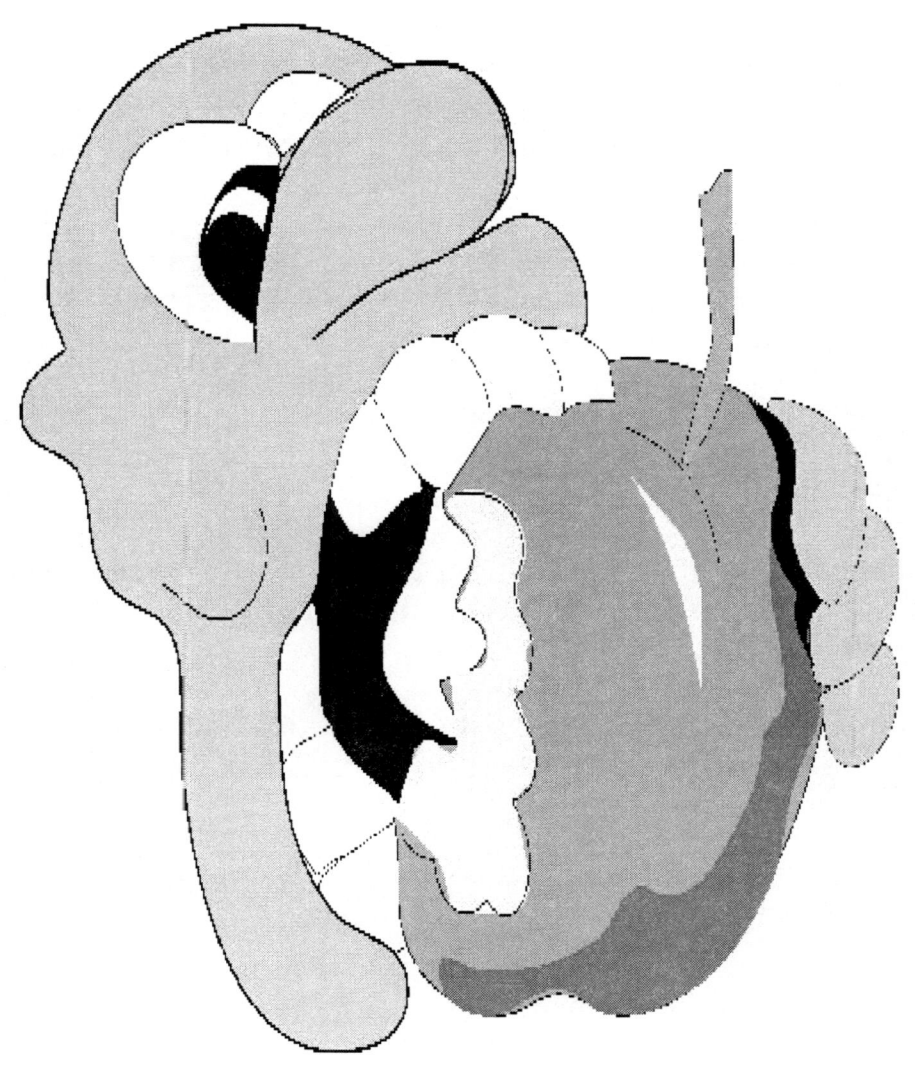

MEAL LIST 3

1 low fat Pre-packaged sandwich.

----

1 homemade sandwich made with 2 slices of wholemeal bread spread with low fat spread and filled with 2oz of wafer thin ham.

----

1 homemade sandwich made with 2 slices of wholemeal bread spread with low fat spread and filled with 2oz of wafer thin chicken.

----

1 homemade sandwich made with 2 slices of wholemeal bread spread with low fat spread and filled with 2oz of canned sardines in tomato sauce.

----

1 homemade sandwich made with 2 slices of wholemeal bread spread with low fat spread and filled with 2oz of wafer thin smoked ham.

----

1 homemade sandwich made with 2 slices of wholemeal bread spread with low fat spread and filled with 2oz of wafer thin pastrami.

----

1 homemade sandwich made with 2 slices of wholemeal bread spread with low fat spread and filled with 2oz of canned salmon.

----

1 homemade sandwich made with 2 slices of wholemeal bread spread with low fat spread and filled with 2oz of prawns.

----

1 homemade sandwich made with 2 slices of wholemeal bread spread with low fat spread with any filling.

MEAL LIST 3

Salad of lettuce, cucumber, onion, tomato, grated carrot plus 6 oz of Prawns and one tablespoon of Kraft Fat Free Thousand Island dressing.

Salad of lettuce, cucumber, onion, tomato, grated carrot plus 6oz of Shrimps and one tablespoon of Kraft Fat Free Thousand Island dressing.

Salad of lettuce, cucumber, onion, tomato, grated carrot plus 8oz of Cottage cheese one tablespoon of Crosse & Blackwell Waistline Low Fat Vinaigrette dressing.

Salad of lettuce, cucumber, onion, tomato, grated carrot plus 4oz of Turkey one tablespoon of Crosse & Blackwell Waistline Low Fat Vinaigrette dressing.

----

1 Slimmers Cup-a-Soup plus 4 Ryvitas spread with 4oz of cottage cheese plus .

----

1 Slimmers Cup-a-Soup plus 4 Ryvitas spread with 4oz of low fat soft cheese plus .

----

1 Slimmers Cup-a-Soup plus 4 Ryvitas spread with low fat spread and top with 2oz of wafer thin smoked ham plus 1 piece of fruit.

----

1 Slimmers Cup-a-Soup plus 4 Ryvitas spread with 4oz of diet coleslaw plus .

----

1 Slimmers Cup-a-Soup plus 4 Ryvitas spread with low fat spread and top with 2oz of wafer thin turkey plus .

MEAL LIST 3

1 homemade sandwich made with 2 slices of wholemeal bread spread with low fat spread and filled with 2oz of mackerel.

----

1 homemade sandwich made with 2 slices of wholemeal bread spread with low fat spread and filled with 3oz of low fat cottage cheese.

----

1 Slimmers Cup-a-Soup plus 2 Ryvitas spread with 4oz of cottage cheese.

----

1 Slimmers Cup-a-Soup plus 2 Ryvitas spread with 2oz of low fat soft cheese.

----

1 Slimmers Cup-a-Soup plus 2 Ryvitas spread with low fat spread and top with 2oz of wafer thin smoked ham.

----

1 Slimmers Cup-a-Soup plus 2 Ryvitas spread with 2oz of diet coleslaw.

----

1 Slimmers Cup-a-Soup plus 2 Ryvitas spread with low fat spread and top with 2 oz of wafer thin turkey.

----

1 Slimmers Cup-a-Soup plus 2 Ryvitas spread with low fat spread and top with 2 oz of wafer thin chicken.

----

1 Heinz Lunchbowls Beef Curry with Rice.

----

1 Findus Lean Cuisine Snackpots Risotto Milanese.

1 Heinz Lunchbowls Country Vegetable Casserole plus .

MEAL LIST 3

1 Heinz Lunchbowls Chicken Curry with Rice.

----

1 Heinz Lunchbowls Lamb & Vegetable Casserole.

----

1 Findus Lean Cuisine Snackpots Chicken & Broccoli Pasta.

----

1 Findus Lean Cuisine Snackpots Chinese Noodle.

----

1 16oz can of Weight Watchers from Heinz Italian Tortelini.

----

1 Heinz Lunchbowls Beef Curry with Rice.

----

1 Heinz Lunchbowls Chilli Con Carne with Rice.

----

1 Findus Lean Cuisine Snackpots Thai Prawn Rice.

----

1 Findus Lean Cuisine Snackpots Szechuan Chicken Chow Mein.

----

1 Findus Lean Cuisine Snackpots Sweet & Sour Pork.

----

1 Findus Lean Cuisine Snackpots Spanish Paella.

Can of Heinz Big Soup Chicken & Ham.

Can of Heinz Big Soup Chicken with Pasta & Vegetable.

Can of Heinz Big Soup Giant Chicken & Vegetable.

Can of Heinz Big Soup Chicken Leek & Potato.

Can of Heinz Big Soup Lamb & Vegetable.

MEAL LIST 3

Can of Heinz Big Soup Chicken & Ham.

Can of Heinz Big Soup Chicken with Pasta & Vegetable.

Can of Heinz Big Soup Giant Chicken & Vegetable.

Can of Heinz Big Soup Chicken Leek & Potato.

Can of Heinz Big Soup Lamb & Vegetable.

----

1 McVites Go-Ahead Apple Bake.

----

1 McVites Go-Ahead Apple Fruit-In.

----

1 McVites Go-Ahead Apricot Fruit-In.

----

1 Boots Breakfast Bar.

----

1 Boots Shapers Apple and Sultana Cereal Bar.

----

1 Boots Shapers Apricot and Chocolate Chip Cereal Bar.

----

1 Jacob's Club Fruit.

----

1 Lo Crazy Caramel Bar.

----

1 Lo Magic Mint.

----

1 Lo White Chocolate.

----

1 Lo Max.

MEAL LIST 4

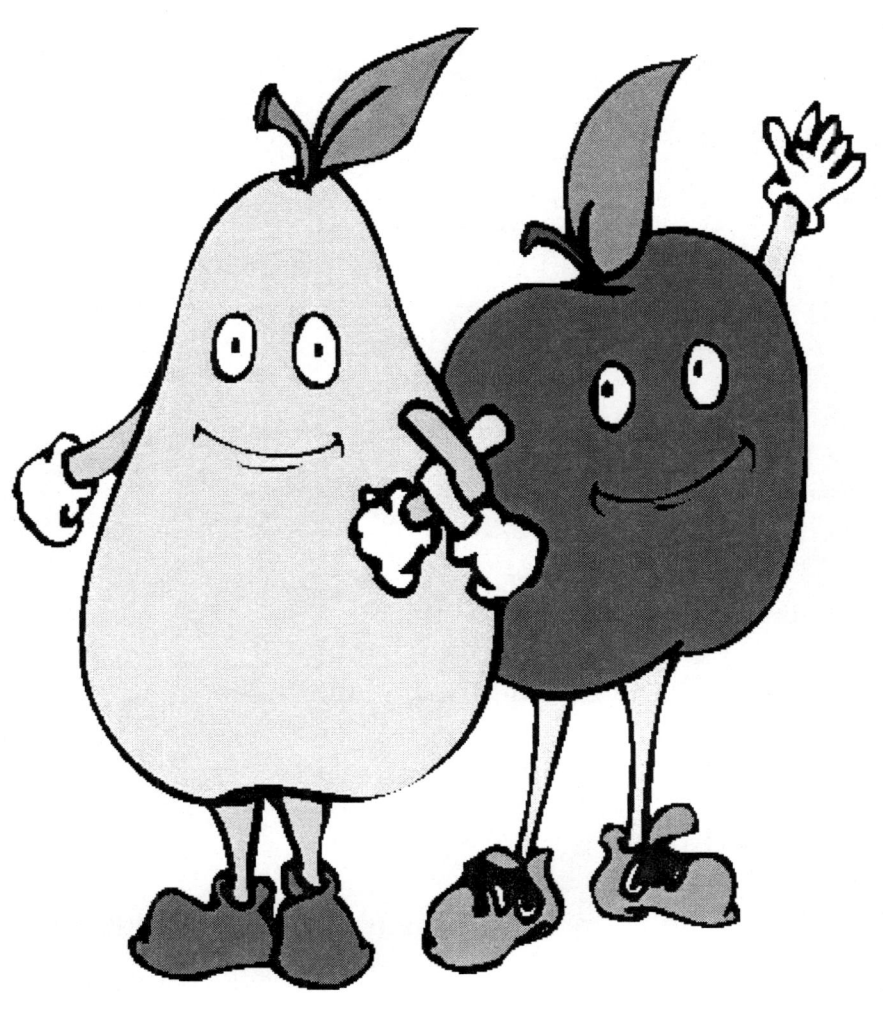

MEAL LIST 4

1 7oz jacket potato filled with 4oz of low fat cottage cheese with pineapple or chives and a salad and one tablespoon of Crosse & Blackwell Waistline Low Fat Vinaigrette dressing.

----

1 7oz jacket potato filled with a jar of potato toppers chicken & vegetable and a salad and one tablespoon of Crosse & Blackwell Waistline Low Fat Vinaigrette dressing.

----

1 16oz can of Weight Watchers from Heinz Italian Vegetable Ravioli.

----

1 Heinz Lunchbowls Chilli Con Carne with Rice.

----

1 Heinz Lunchbowls Spaghetti Bolognese.

----

1 Findus Lean Cuisine Snackpots Risotto Milanese.

----

1 16oz can of Weight Watchers from Heinz Italian Tuna Twists.

Can of Heinz Big Soup Beef & Bacon.

Can of Heinz Big Soup Giant Beef Bolognese.

Can of Heinz Big Soup Beef Broth.

Can of Heinz Big Soup Beef & Vegetable.

Can of Heinz Big Soup Thick Country Vegetable with Ham.

----

1 Findus Lean Cuisine Snackpots Smoked Ham & Mushroom Tagliatlle.

MEAL LIST 4

Can of Heinz Big Soup Giant Minestrone plus

----

1 7oz jacket potato filled with a jar of potato toppers chicken & vegetable and a salad.

----

1 16oz can of Weight Watchers from Heinz Italian Tuna Twists

----

1 16oz can of Weight Watchers from Heinz Italian Tortelin

----

1 16oz can of Weight Watchers from Heinz Italian Vegetable Ravioli

----

1 Findus Lean Cuisine Snackpots Vegetable Balti.

Can of Heinz Big Soup Spicy Tomato with Beef Pasta Parcels.

Salad of lettuce, cucumber, onion, tomato, grated carrot plus 6oz of Prawns and one tablespoon of Kraft Fat Free Thousand Island dressing.

----

1 Linda Mc-Cartney Ploughman's Pasty.

----

1 Linda Mc-Cartney Deep Pies.

----

1 Linda Mc-Cartney Potato Wedges.

----

1 Linda Mc-Cartney Stew and Dumplings.

----

1 Linda Mc-Cartney Creamy Cajum Bake.

----

1 Linda Mc-Cartney Chilli Con Carne.

MEAL LIST 4

Salad of lettuce, cucumber, onion, tomato, grated carrot plus 6oz of Shrimps and one tablespoon of Kraft Fat Free Thousand Island dressing.

Salad of lettuce, cucumber, onion, tomato, grated carrot plus 6oz of Lobster and one tablespoon of Kraft Fat Free Thousand Island dressing.

Salad of lettuce, cucumber, onion, tomato, grated carrot plus 6oz of Crab and one tablespoon of Kraft Fat Free Thousand Island dressing.

Salad of lettuce, cucumber, onion, tomato, grated carrot plus 5oz of Chicken breast one tablespoon of Crosse & Blackwell Waistline Low Fat Vinaigrette dressing

----

Salad of lettuce, cucumber, onion, tomato, grated carrot plus 4oz of Turkey one tablespoon of Crosse & Blackwell Waistline Low Fat Vinaigrette dressing.

Salad of lettuce, cucumber, onion, tomato, grated carrot plus 4oz of Cheese one tablespoon of Crosse & Blackwell Waistline Low Fat Vinaigrette dressing.

Salad of lettuce, cucumber, onion, tomato, grated carrot plus 4oz of Ham one tablespoon of Low Fat Vinaigrette dressing.

Salad of lettuce, cucumber, onion, tomato, grated carrot plus 8oz of Cottage cheese one tablespoon of Crosse & Blackwell Waistline Low Fat Vinaigrette dressing.

MEAL LIST 5

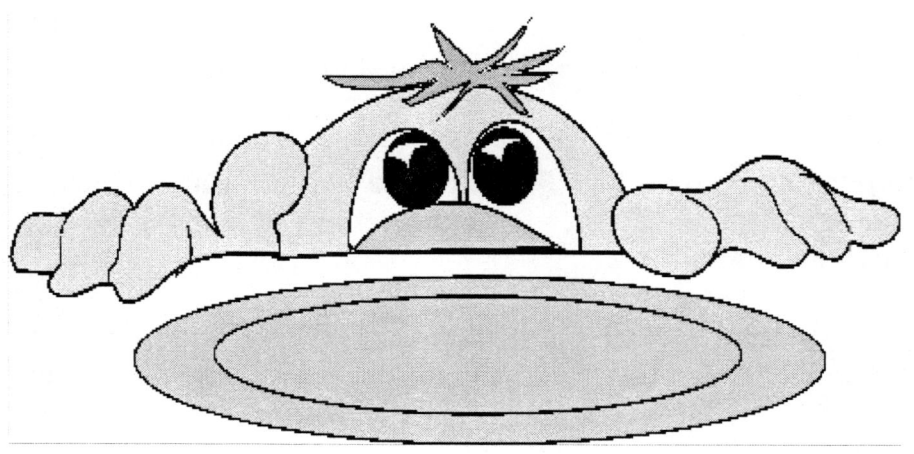

MEAL LIST 5

Birds Eye Cod Steak in Butter Sauce served with 4oz of potatoes either fresh or any instant mash mix, 7oz of any vegetables.

Birds Eye Cod Steak in Parsley Sauce served with 4oz of potatoes either fresh or any instant mash mix, 7oz of any vegetables.

Iceland Salmon in Lemon & Herb Sauce served with 4oz of potatoes either fresh or any instant mash mix, 7oz of any vegetables.

One portion of Birds Eye Fish Cuisine Italiano Bake served with 4oz of potatoes either fresh or any instant mash mix, 7oz of any vegetables.

One tin of John West Tuna in Thousand Island served with 4oz of potatoes a salad of lettuce, cucumber, onion, tomato, grated carrot plus one tablespoon of C & B waistline low fat vinaigrette.

One tin of John West Tuna in Mayonnaise & Sweetcorn served with 4oz of potatoes a salad of lettuce, cucumber, onion, tomato, grated carrot plus one tablespoon of C & B waistline low fat vinaigrette.

Harry Ramsdens Giant Cod Cake served with 4oz of oven chips or 4oz of potatoes either fresh or any instant mash mix, and 7oz of any vegetables.

MEAL LIST 5

Harry Ramsdens Ovenbake Cod Steak served with 4oz of oven chips or 4oz of potatoes either fresh or any instant mash mix, and 7oz of any vegetables.

Harry Ramsdens Ovenbake Haddock Steak served with 4oz of oven chips or 4oz of potatoes either fresh or any instant mash mix, and 7oz of any vegetables.

One Ross Cod Dog in a bun served with 4oz of oven chips a salad of lettuce, cucumber, onion, tomato, grated carrot plus one tablespoon of C & B waistline low fat vinaigrette.

One tin of John West Tuna in Curry Sauce served with 4oz of potatoes a Salad of lettuce, cucumber, onion, tomato, grated carrot plus one tablespoon of C & B waistline low fat vinaigrette.

One portion of Birds Eye Fish Cuisine Mushroom Parisienne Bake served with 4oz of potatoes either fresh or any instant mash mix, 7oz of any vegetables.

Iceland Haddock Fillet in a Creamy Cheese Sauce served with 4oz of potatoes either fresh or any instant mash mix, 7oz of any vegetables.

Iceland Cod Steak in Mushroom & White Wine Sauce served with 4oz of potatoes either fresh or any instant mash mix, 7oz of any vegetables.

----

1 Slimmers Cup-a-Soup plus 4 Ryvitas spread with low fat spread and top with 2oz of wafer thin turkey.

MEAL LIST 5

Birds Eye Cod Steak in Mushroom Sauce served with 4oz of potatoes either fresh or any instant mash mix, 7oz of any vegetables.

Iceland Cod Steak in Butter Sauce served with 4oz of potatoes either fresh or any instant mash mix, 7oz of any vegetables.

One portion of Birds Eye Fish Cuisine Garlic Bordelaise Crumb Bake served with 4oz of potatoes either fresh or any instant mash mix, 7oz of any vegetables.

One portion of Birds Eye Fish Cuisine Vegetable Tuscany Bake served with 4oz of potatoes either fresh or any instant mash mix, 7oz of any vegetables.

One tin of John West Tuna In Mayonnaise Garlic & Herbs served with 4oz of potatoes a salad of lettuce, cucumber, onion, tomato, grated carrot plus one tablespoon of C & B waistline vinaigrette.

One Tesco Healthy Eating Breaded Cod served with 4oz of oven chips and 7oz of any vegetables

----

Birds Eye Chicken Lattice Cheddar Cheese & Broccoli Flavour served with 4oz of potatoes either fresh or any instant mash mix, 7oz of any vegetables.

Birds Eye Chicken Marinade Spicy Cajun Flavour served with 4oz of potatoes either fresh or any instant mash mix, 7oz of any vegetables.

MEAL LIST 5

Birds Eye Chicken in a Creamy Garlic & Herb Sauce served with 4oz of potatoes either fresh or any instant mash mix, 7oz of any vegetables.

Weight Watchers from Heinz Chicken Korma with Rice plus .

Weight Watchers from Heinz Lamb Moussaka served with 7oz of any vegetables.

Two of Tesco Healthy Eating Pork Kebabs served with 4oz of chilled saffron rice.

One 8oz of Tesco Healthy Eating Pork Leg Steak with 4oz of potatoes either fresh or any instant mash mix, 7oz of any vegetables.

Birds Eye Chicken Lattice Creamy Mushroom Flavour served with 4oz of potatoes either fresh or any instant mash mix, 7oz of any vegetables.

Birds Eye Chicken Marinade French Garlic & Herb Flavour served with 4oz of potatoes either fresh or any instant mash mix, 7oz of any vegetables.

Birds Eye Chicken in a Creamy Curry Sauce served with 4oz of chilled saffron rice.

Weight Watchers from Heinz Chicken & Broccoli Pasta Bake served with 7oz of any vegetables.

Weight Watchers from Heinz Shepherd's Pie with Lamb served with 7oz of any vegetables.

MEAL LIST 5

1 7oz jacket potato filled with 4oz of low fat cottage cheese with pineapple or chives and a salad and one tablespoon of Crosse & Blackwell Waistline Low Fat Vinaigrette dressing.

----

1 7oz jacket potato filled with 4oz of sweetcorn and a salad and one tablespoon of Crosse & Blackwell Waistline Low Fat Vinaigrette dressing

----

1 7oz jacket potato filled with a 6oz can of baked beans.

----

1 7oz jacket potato filled with a jar of potato toppers chicken & vegetable and a salad and one tablespoon of Crosse & Blackwell Waistline Low Fat Vinaigrette dressing.

----

1 16oz can of Weight Watchers from Heinz Italian Tuna Twists.

----

1 16oz can of Weight Watchers from Heinz Italian Tortelini.

----

1 Heinz Lunchbowls Beef Curry with Rice.

----

1 Heinz Lunchbowls Chicken Curry with Rice.

----

1 Heinz Lunchbowls Spaghetti Bolognese.

----

1 Findus Lean Cuisine Snackpots Arabiatta.

----

1 Findus Lean Cuisine Snackpots Chicken & Broccoli Pasta.

----

1 Findus Lean Cuisine Snackpots Risotto Milanese.

----

1 Findus Lean Cuisine Snackpots Chicken & Prawn Creole.

MEAL LIST 5

1 Findus Lean Cuisine Snackpots Chinese Noodle.

----

1 low fat Pre-packaged sandwiches.

One box of Honey Nut Shredded Wheat from Nestle Pic-a-Pac with milk taken from the daily allowance

----

1 slice of wholemeal bread toasted with 2 teaspoons of marmalade or jam.

----

2 cooked turkey rashers 2 slices of wholemeal bread toasted and spread with low fat spread.

----

1 whole fresh pink grapefruit and a boiled egg with a slice of wholemeal bread spread with low fat spread.

----

1 slice of wholemeal bread toasted and spread with low fat spread top with a 7oz / 200g can of heated tomatoes and a cooked turkey rasher.

----

2 slice of wholemeal bread toasted and spread with low fat spread top with a cooked turkey rasher 7oz tin of mushrooms. Weight Watchers from Heinz Vegetable & Pasta Medley served with 7oz of any vegetables.

Weight Watchers from Heinz Chilled Meals Vegetable Chilli enchiladas with Naan bread served 4oz of chilled saffron rice.

Tesco chilled meals Vegetable Curry served 4oz of chilled saffron rice.

MEAL LIST 5

Linda Mc-Cartney Lasagne served with 4oz of potatoes either fresh or any instant mash mix, 7oz of any vegetables.

One Linda Mc-Cartney Stew & Dumpling served with 4oz of potatoes either fresh or any instant mash mix, 7oz of any vegetables.

½ of Bachelors Beanfast Bolognese style mix served with 4oz of potatoes either fresh or any instant mash mix, or 4oz of cooked pasta.

½ of Bachelors Beanfast Savoury Mince style mix served with 4oz of potatoes either fresh or any instant mash mix.

Weight Watchers from Heinz Vegetable Hotpot served with 7oz of any vegetables.

Weight Watchers from Heinz Vegetable Stroganoff served with 7oz of any vegetables.

Tesco Chilled Meals Harvest Vegetable Pie served with 7oz of any vegetables.

Salad of lettuce, cucumber, onion, tomato, grated carrot plus 6 oz of Prawns and one tablespoon of Kraft Fat Free Thousand Island dressing.

Salad of lettuce, cucumber, onion, tomato, grated carrot plus 6oz of Shrimps and one tablespoon of Kraft Fat Free Thousand Island dressing.

Getting Out of the Kitchen

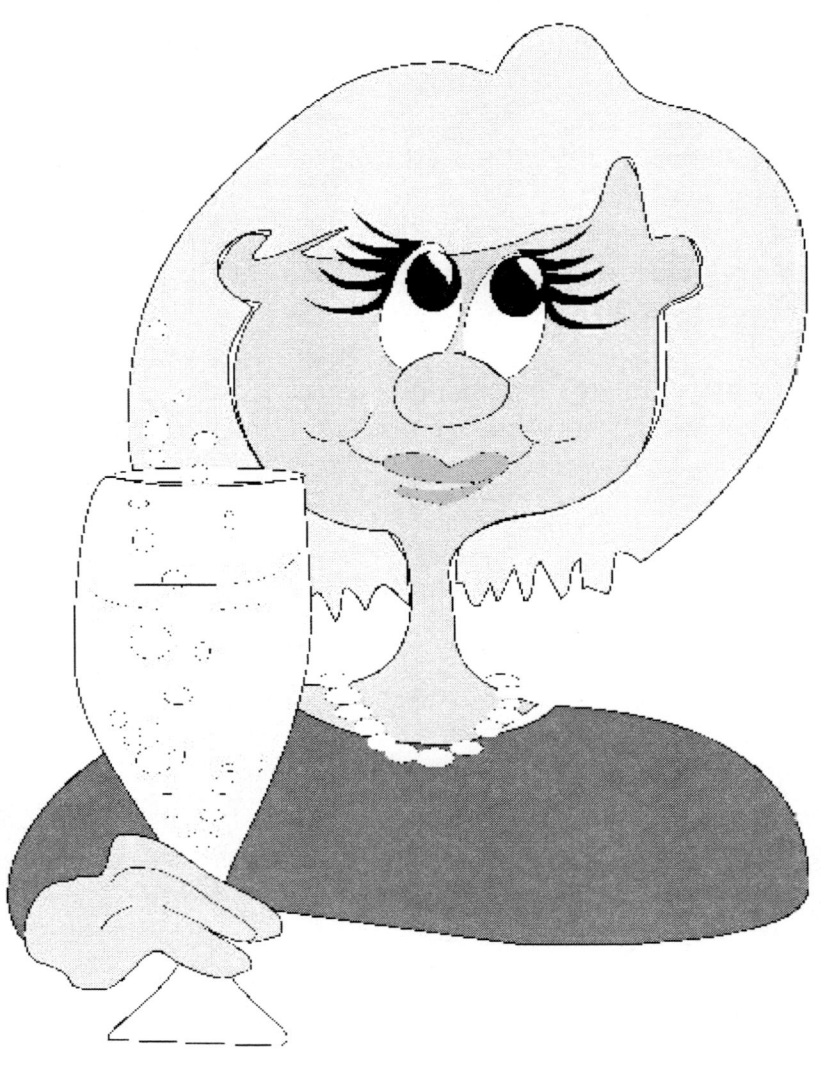

Getting Out of the Kitchen

Eating healthily does not have to mean you spending hours in the kitchen.

- Organise your time were possible try to plan meals in advance and write a details shopping list and only what's on the list not what's on offer at the shops.

- Before cooking a meal get all the necessary ingredients together.
- Scrub vegetables rather then peel were possible as this will not only save you time but will add extra fibre to your meals.

- Try to use one-pot recipes such as soups, casseroles and stir-fries and try to use only non-stick pots. Because it not only saves you time with the washing up but money on the fuel you use to cook the food.

- If you have a microwave oven make full use of it do not just use for heating food up.

- Frozen vegetables are quicker to cook and are an alternative to fresh.

- If you have a freeze why not prepare dishes in advance then freeze for when you just want a lazy meal.

- If you keep a good stock of convenience foods they will be at hand so you do not miss a meal when you are busy.

Convenience foods products do not be junk foods if you try and keep these in you store cupboard or freezer for a standby.

- Canned baked beans and tins of spaghetti.

- Lean Cuisine Snackpots meals.

- Heinz Lunchbowls.

- Meat free ravioli.

- Meat free spaghetti Bolognese.

- Canned tuna in brine.

- Mealmakers tuna Bolognese.

- Mealmakers tuna chilli.

- Mealmakers tuna supreme.

- Canned salmon.

- Canned sardines in brine.

- Cans of Heinz Big soup.

- Jar of Potato Toppers.

- Weight Watchers from Heinz canned Italian Foods.

- Canned tomatoes.

- Canned fruit in natural juices.

- Any ready meals.

Recipes

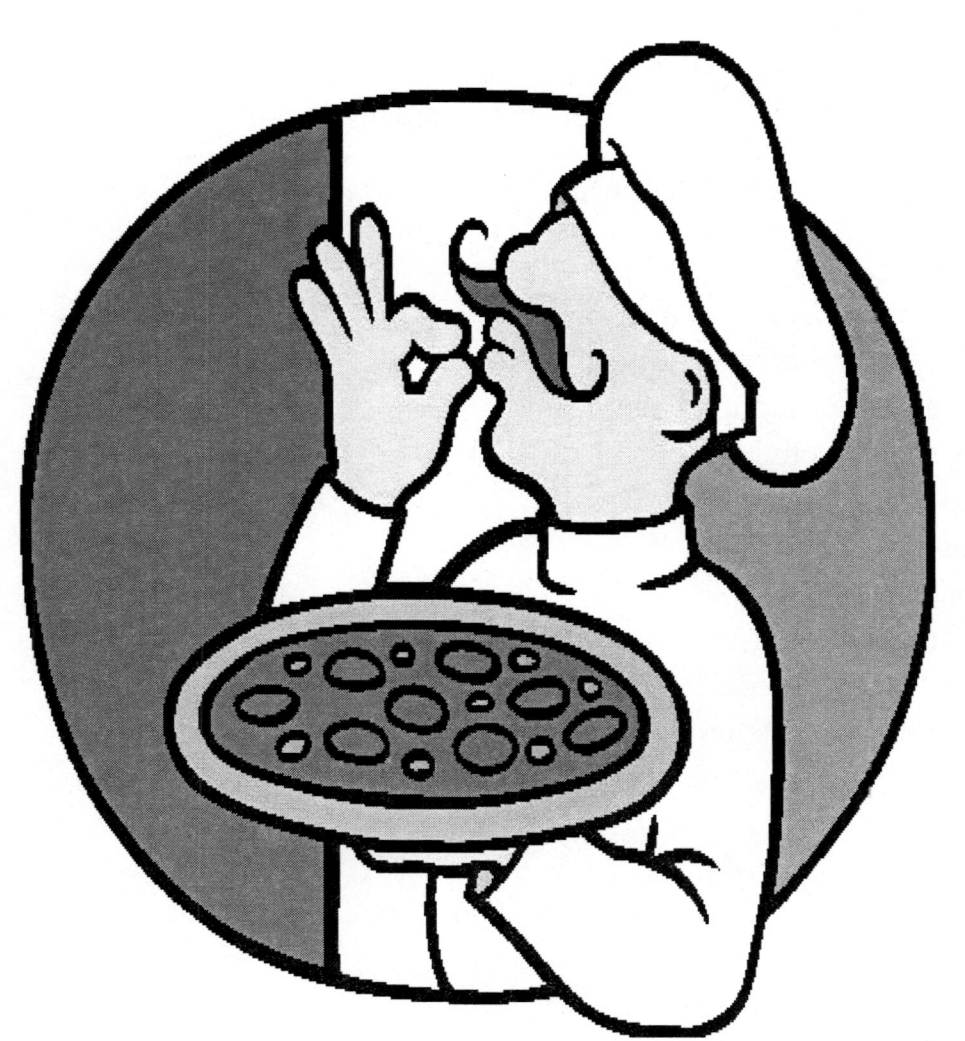

Recipes

This is a collection of basic recipes that have been created just for one for when you needs to cook just a single meal. All the recipes have been designed to use the basic of cooking utensils.

Find there are 2 or more of you no problem just multiply the ingredients by how many of you there are it is that simple. Cooking without kitchen scales all that is needed for these recipes is a set of measuring spoons and measuring cups.

Breakfasts

Light Meals

Main Meals

Snacks and Suppers

Puddings

Breakfasts

Bacon & Cheese Crumpet

1	Rasher	Bacon
1	medium	Crumpet
1	Slice	Cheddar Cheese

1. Grill the rasher of bacon until it is cooked.
2. Warm the crumpet and cut in half leaving a hinged side.
3. Place cooked bacon on one side and the sliced cheese on the other.
4. Return to grill until the cheese is just melting and crumpet is only lightly toasted then close and eat at once.

Bacon & Cheese with Herbs Croissant

1	Rasher	Bacon
1	Medium	Croissant
2	Tablespoon	Low Fat Soft Cheese with Herbs

1. Grill the rasher of bacon until it is cooked.
2. Cut the croissant in half leaving a hinged side.
3. Toast croissant until it is a light golden brown.
4. Place cooked bacon on one side and spread the low fat soft cheese with herbs on the other, close and eat at once.

Banana & Orange Breakfast Shake

2	Cups	Milk
1	Medium	Banana
½	Cup	Orange Juice
5		Ice Cubes
1	Teaspoon	Wheat germ
3	Drops	Vanilla Extract

1. Peeled and sliced the banana.

2. Combine all the ingredients in a blender container.

3. Blend until smooth, about 20 seconds.

Serving Suggestion
Pour into a glass and drink at once.

Banana Delight

1	Cup	Banana Yoghurt
1	Medium	Banana
5	Whole	Ice Cubes
2	Cups	Milk
1	Teaspoon	Wheat germ
3	Drops	Vanilla Extract

1. Peeled and sliced the banana.
2. Combine all the ingredients in a blender container.
3. Blend until smooth, about 20 seconds.

Serving Suggestion
Pour into a glass and drink at once.

Hot Scrambled Eggs

2	Medium	Eggs
1	Small	Onion, chopped very finely
1	Tablespoon	Butter
1	Teaspoon	Tomato Puree
1	Teaspoon	Curry Powder
1	Slice	Bread

1. Place a pan over a moderate heat add butter and melt add curry powder and onions cook until they are soft, about 10 minutes.

2. Break the eggs into a bowl add the tomato puree and beat.

3. Add egg mix to pan and stir then reduce to a low heat.

4. Stir occasionally until eggs are set.

5. Toast bread under grill and pour eggs on top.

Jugged Kipper

1   Whole   Fresh Kipper
1   Large Jug   Boiling Water

1. Place the kipper in a large jug.
2. Pour the boiling water over it so the tail is just uncovered.
3. Leave for 5 minutes then remove.
4. Place on warm plate and top with a knob of butter

Curried Eggs

2	Medium	Eggs, hard-boiled and quartered
2	Tablespoons	Butter
1	Teaspoon	Curry Powder
1	Tablespoon	Water
1	Pinch	Salt & Pepper

1. Place a pan over a moderate heat and add butter and melt, then add eggs, curry power, salt and pepper and water stir carefully.

2. Cook for 2 minutes only.

3. To serve just pour on to a hot plate.

Grapefruit Surprise

1   Medium   Grapefruit
1   Tablespoon   Sugar
1   Tablespoon   Port

1. Cut grapefruit in half loosen segments with a knife and remove any pips.
2. Place one half in an ovenproof dish sprinkle with sugar and pour the port over the top.
3. Place under a hot grill for a few minutes until the sugar melts and turns brown.

Serving Suggestion
Remove and serve at once.

Quick Kedgeree

½	Cup	Cooked White Rice
½	Cup	Cooked smoked haddock, flaked
1	Medium	Hard Boiled Egg, chopped
1	Tablespoon	Evaporated Milk
1	Tablespoon	Turmeric
½	Teaspoon	Nutmeg, grated

1. Mix all the ingredients in a bowl except the oil.
2. Heat a frying pan over a moderate heat and the oil then empty the bowl into the pan and warm for about 3 to 5 minutes.

Serving Suggestion
Serve on a warm plate

Strawberry Delight

1	Cup	Strawberry Yoghurt
1	Cup	Canned Strawberries
2	Cups	Milk
5	Whole	Ice Cubes
1	Teaspoon	Wheat germ
3	Drops	Vanilla Extract

1. Combine all the ingredients in blender container.
2. Blend until smooth, about 20 seconds.
3. Pour into a glass and drink at once.

Light Meals

Beef Risotto

1	Cup	Diced Cooked Beef
½	Cup	Italian Risotto Rice
2	Cups	Water
1	Small	Chopped Tomato
1	Small	Onion
1	Medium	Yellow Pepper
1	Medium	Green Pepper
1		Beef Stock Cube
1	Tablespoon	Extra Virgin Olive Oil
½	Teaspoon	Salt & Pepper

1. Peel and very finely chop the onion.

2. Chop the peppers and tomato.

3. Heat a saucepan and melt the butter and add the chopped onion, peppers and tomato, sauté for 2 to 3 minutes until they have softened.

4. Now add herbs and rice to pan stir well and cook for another 1 minute.

5. Mix stock cube with water and add to saucepan.

6. Add the stock, tomato, beef, salt and pepper to the pan and bring to the boil.

7. Reduce the heat and simmer for 12 to 15 minutes until all the water has been absorbed and the rice is cooked.

8. To serve pour onto a warm plate and eat at once.

Broccoli Lasagne

4	Sheets	Lasagne
½	Cup	Creamed Cottage Cheese
2	Cups	Frozen Broccoli
½	Cup	Natural Yoghurt
¼	Cup	Mozzarella Cheese, grated
1	Tablespoon	Yoghurt
1	Pinch	Salt & Pepper

1. Place broccoli into a pan of boiling water and cook for 5 minutes and then drain.

2. Mix cottage cheese natural yoghurt, salt and pepper in a bowl then add the broccoli.

3. In an ovenproof dish place a quarter of the broccoli mix then cover with one sheet of lasagne

4. Repeat this twice.

5. Now add last of mix and sprinkle with the mozzarella cheese.

6. Cover tightly with aluminium foil bake in a moderate oven at 350°F, 180 °C or Gas Mark 4, for 30 minutes or until cheese melts and is golden on top.

7. Remove from the oven and serve on a warm plate, eat at once.

Cauliflower Cheese

3	Cups	Cauliflower Florets
1	Tablespoon	Butter
½	Cup	Grated Cheddar Cheese
1	Dash	Worcestershire Sauce

1. Put the cauliflower in a pot of boiling salted water and cook for 12 minutes.

2. Drain the cauliflower and return to pot.

3. Add butter and stir until melted over a low heat.

4. Then add cheese, stirring it constantly, until cheese melts.

5. Season with a dash of Worcestershire sauce.

6. Serve at once on a warm plate.

Serving Suggestion
Try serving with a tomato salad and a whole-wheat roll.

Celery Soufflé

½ Small Tin   Celery
½ Small Tin   Condensed Celery Soup
1   Large   Egg
1   Pinch   Salt & Pepper

1. Grease a small soufflé dish and empty in the celery.
2. Separate the egg.
3. Empty the celery soup into a bowl and add the egg yolk, salt and pepper and mix together well.
4. Then whisk the egg white until it is stiff fold into egg yolk mixture.
5. Pour over celery and bake at 400°F, 200°C or Gas Mark 6 for 20 to 25 minutes until golden brown.
6. Serve at once on a warm plate.

Serving Suggestion
Try serving with a tomato salad and a whole-wheat roll.

Cheese & Mushroom Rolls

2	Sheets	Filo Pastry
2	Tablespoons	Warmed Extra Virgin Olive Oil
½	Cup	Grated Cheddar Cheese
1	Medium	Chopped Mushroom
1	Teaspoon	Lime Juice
½	Teaspoon	Mixed Herbs

1. Lay out flat one of the sheets of filo pastry and brush with oil then brush the other sheet with oil and place over the top of the first one.

2. Mix together the mushrooms, tomatoes, lime juice and herbs.

3. Place in the middle of the sheets and spread out.

4. Now start at one end and roll up the filo pastry.

5. Transfer to an oiled baking sheet and brush with oil.

6. Bake in a moderate oven at 375°F, 190°C or Gas Mark 5 for 12 to 18 minutes till golden brown.

7. Remove from the oven and serve at once on a warm plate.

Main Meals

Baked Cajun Fish

1	Tablespoon	Fresh White Breadcrumbs
1	Tablespoon	Chopped Fresh Parsley
1	Clove	Garlic, crushed
1	Pinch	Salt & Pepper
1	Teaspoon	Cajun Seasoning
1	Teaspoon	Lemon Zest
1	Tablespoon	Extra Virgin Olive Oil
1	Portion	White Fish Fillet

1. In a shallow dish mix together the breadcrumbs, parsley; salt, pepper, Cajun seasoning, lemon zest and crushed garlic.

2. Preheat oven to 325°F, 160°C or Gas Mark 3.

3. Brush the fish fillet on both sides with the olive oil; and then dip into the breadcrumb mixture making sure to coat both sides well.

4. Butter a baking dish and place fish into it and cover with a sheet of tin foil.

5. Bake for 10 to 12 minutes, then remove foil and cook for a further 2 to 3 minutes to let fish brown.

6. Remove fish from the oven and serve at once.

Beef Lasagne

2	Sheets	No Pre-Cooking Lasagne
1	Small Tin	Chopped Tomatoes,
2	Cups	Lean Minced Beef
2	Cloves	Garlic
1	Small	Onion
2	Tablespoons	Grated Mozzarella Cheese,
1	Teaspoon	Tomato Puree
1	Teaspoon	Italian Seasoning
1	Tablespoon	Butter
2	Cups	Milk
1	Tablespoon	Cornflour

1. Heat a frying pan over a moderate heat and add the beef stir until meat browns and separates into grains.

2. Peel and finely chop the onion and crush the garlic, add to the frying pan with the chopped tomatoes, tomato puree and Italian seasoning.

3. Bring to the boil then reduce heat cook for about 14 to 18 minutes until sauce thickens.

4. Put half of the mixture into a shallow ovenproof dish cover with a sheet of lasagne then the remaining sauces and top with a sheet of lasagne.

5. Place a pan over a medium heat add the butter and melt then add the cornflour and cook for 1 to 2 minutes stirring all the time.

6. Slowly add the milk, salt and pepper, stir well and increase the heat and cook for 4 minutes until sauce thickens.

7. Pour over the top of the last sheet of lasagne and sprinkle with the Mozzarella Cheese.

8. Bake in a moderate oven at 375°F, 190 °C or Gas Mark 5 for 25 to 30 minutes till golden brown.

Beef Stroganoff

1	Portion	Beef Fillet Steak
2	Tablespoons	Butter
1	Small	Onion, thinly sliced
1	Cup	Button Mushrooms
1	Tablespoon	Brandy or Schnapps
¼	Cup	Cream
1	Pinch	Salt & Pepper

1. Cut steak into thin strips about an inch long.

2. Heat a fry pan and add 1 tablespoon of the butter.

3. Add onions and sauté for 2 to 3 minutes until softened.

4. Now add mushrooms to pan and sauté them both for a further 2 minutes.

5. Remove from pan now add remaining butter to pan and melt.

6. Add beef and sauté for about 3 to 5 minutes.

7. Now add brandy to beef in pan and ignite shake pan until flames subside.

8. Return mushrooms and onions to pan add salt, pepper and stir in cream.

9. Cook for about 1 minute until all the ingredients are well heated.

Serving Suggestion
To serve pour onto a warm plate and eat at once.

Bolognese

2	Cups	Lean Minced Beef
1	Small	Finely Chopped Onion
1	Small Tin	Chopped Tomatoes
1	Teaspoon	Tomato Puree
2	Cloves	Garlic
1	Teaspoon	Italian Seasoning
1	Portion	Spaghetti
1	Tablespoon	Parmesan Cheese

1. Heat a frying pan over a moderate heat and add the beef and onions.

2. Crush the garlic and add it to the frying pan, stir until meat browns and separates into grains.

3. Add chopped tomatoes, tomato puree and Italian seasoning.

4. Bring to the boil then reduce heat stiring from time to time.

5. Cook for about 14 to 18 minutes until sauce thickens.

6. Cook the spaghetti according to the directions on the packet.

7. When cooked drain and put on plate spoon the bolognese sauce over it and top with Parmesan cheese.

Chicken Kebabs

1	Medium	Chicken Breast, cubed
1	Medium	Red Pepper, cubed
8	Small	Button Mushrooms
2	Tablespoons	Natural Yoghurt
1	Teaspoon	Curry Paste
1	Pinch	Salt & Pepper
2	Cloves	Garlic, crushed

1. Place cubed chicken breast, mushrooms and peppers in to a bowl with the honey, yoghurt, garlic, seasoning and curry paste mix together.

2. Assemble kebab by pushing chicken onto skewers alternating with the peppers and mushrooms.

3. Cook under a hot grill for 12 to 14 minutes turning frequently.

Serving Suggestion
To serve place on a bed of rice.

Snacks and Suppers

Scrambled Egg Pockets

1	Cup	Tinned Tomatoes, chopped
1	Small	Onion, chopped
1	Small	Green Bell Pepper, chopped
1	Large	Egg
1	Tablespoon	Extra Virgin Olive Oil
1	Teaspoon	Mixed Herbs
1	Pinch	Salt & Pepper
1	Whole	Garlic Pita Bread

1. Make a pocket in the pita bread by cutting down one edge.

2. Heat a fry pan and add oil.

3. Add onions and peppers and sauté for 5 to 6 minutes until softened.

4. Now add, tomatoes to pan and sauté for a further 2 minutes.

5. Then add herbs, salt and pepper to egg and beat then pour into pan and stir until set.

6. Spoon the egg mixture into the pita bread pocket.

Serving Suggestion
Serve at once on a warm plate.

Smoked Haddock on Toast

1	Portion	Finnan Haddock
1	Tablespoon	Butter
1	Cup	Milk
1	Tablespoon	Flour
1	Slice	Bread, toasted
1	Pinch	Salt & Pepper

1. Add the milk and butter to saucepan, place over a moderate heat and add fish and cook for 5 to 6 minutes.

2. Remove fish and flake it into dish removing any bones or skin keep warm.

3. Blend the flour with a little milk taken from the saucepan then add to rest of milk and stir.

4. Bring to a boil add salt, pepper and stir the mixture until sauce thickens about 3 to 4 minutes.

5. Toast the bread and butter it then top with the flaked fish pour sauce over the top and serve.

Swiss Eggs

2	Large	Eggs
1	Tablespoon	Butter, grated
1	Tablespoon	Parmesan cheese, grated
1	Tablespoon	Double Cream
1	Tablespoon	Gruyere Cheese, grated
1	Pinch	Parmesan Cheese

1. Butter two ramekins dishes.

2. Break an egg carefully into each cup.

3. Sprinkle with salt and pepper to taste.

4. Pour 1 tablespoon of cream over each egg.

5. Dot eggs with butter and sprinkle with the cheese and pour over cream.

6. Set the ramekins dishes into a baking tin.

7. Now add enough boiling water into baking tin to come half way up the sides of the dishes.

8. Bake in a moderate oven at 350°F, 180°C or Gas Mark 4 for 10 minutes.

Turkey & Cheese Croissant

1	Slice	Cooked Turkey
1		Croissant
1	Slice	Cheddar Cheese

1. Warm the croissant and cut in half leaving a hinged side.
2. Place the slice of turkey on one side and the sliced cheese on the other.
3. Return to grill until the cheese is just melting and croissant is only lightly toasted then close and eat.

Beef Burgers

2	Cups	Lean Minced Beef
1	Cup	Fresh White Breadcrumbs
1	Small	Finely Chopped Onion
1	Teaspoon	Dried Mix Herbs
1	Teaspoon	Tomato Puree

1. In a bowl, mix the onion, beef, breadcrumbs, herbs and tomato puree.
2. Divide the mixture to make two burgers and pat these in to two round shapes.
3. Grill or fry burgers for 10 to 12 minutes turning once.
4. Serve with relish and salad in burger buns.

Bacon & Cheese Pizza

1	Cup	White SR Flour
1	Teaspoon	Salt
1	Tablespoon	Water
2	Tablespoons	Extra Virgin Olive Oil
1	Small	Tin of Chopped Tomatoes
1	Cup	Grated Cheese
1	Rasher	Smoked Bacon
1	Teaspoon	Italian Seasoning

1. In a bowl mix the flour, salt, water and oil to a stiff dough.

2. Roll out the dough on a floured surface into a circle.

3. Then place onto a greased baking sheet.

4. Heat a saucepan over moderate heat add tomatoes and herbs bring to the boil and let boil for 5 to 7 minutes until the sauce has reduced by half then spread over the base.

5. Cover base with the cheese then chop the rasher of bacon and add it.

6. Bake in a moderate oven at 400°F, 200 °C or Gas Mark 6 for 15 to 20 minutes till golden brown.

7. Remove from the oven and serve at once.

Puddings

Almond & White Chocolate Mousse

1	Small	Egg
1	Small Bar	White Chocolate
1	Tablespoon	Sugar
2	Tablespoon	Boiling Water
1	Tablespoon	Chopped Blanched Almonds
1	Teaspoon	Almond Extract

1. Break egg and separate the yolk from the white.

2. Place egg white into a clean medium sized bowl.

3. Now beat egg white until foamy then gradually add the sugar and continue beating until stiff.

4. Place chocolate; egg yolk, boiling water and flavouring into a blender and blend for few seconds until chocolate is melted.

5. Fold chocolate mixture into egg white until no streaks of egg white remain.

6. Turn into a ramekin dish, and chill in a refrigerator for several hours until firm.

7. Remove from the refrigerator and serve at once.

Baked Apple with Brandy

¼	Cup	Glacé Cherries
1	Tablespoon	Brown Sugar
½	Teaspoon	Ground Cinnamon
¼	Teaspoon	Lemon Rind, grated
1	Tablespoon	Brandy
1	Large	Cooking Apple
1	Teaspoon	Clear Honey
2	Cups	Hot Water

1. Combine glacé cherries, brown sugar, cinnamon, lemon rind, and brandy in a small bowl.

2. Core apple three quarters of the way through being careful not to cut through the bottom.

3. Place the apple in a small dish.

4. Fill centre of apples with the mixture and drizzle the honey over top of apple.

5. Set the dish into a baking tin now add enough boiling water into baking tin to come half way up the sides of the dish.

6. During cooking keep basting the apple with syrup from dish and top up the water if needed.

7. Bake in a preheated oven at 400°F, 200°C or Gas Mark 6 for 40 minutes or until tender.

8. Remove from the oven and serve at once.

Serving Suggestion
To serve pour over syrup or try serving with little custard or drizzle with fresh cream.

Banana Delight

1	Cup	Banana Yoghurt
1	Medium	Banana
5	Whole	Ice Cubes
2	Cups	Milk
1	Teaspoon	Wheat germ
3	Drops	Vanilla Extract

1. Peeled and sliced the banana.
2. Combine all the ingredients in a blender container.
3. Blend until smooth, about 20 seconds.

Serving Suggestion
Pour into a glass and drink at once.

Blackcurrant Soufflé

½	Tin	Blackcurrants in Syrup
1	Teaspoon	Sugar
1	Medium	Egg
1	Tablespoon	Butter
1	Tablespoon	SR Flour

1. Place a saucepan over a low heat add the butter and melt with a wooden spoon stir in the flour and cook for 2 minutes.

2. Now slowly add the fruit to the saucepan stir with a whisk until the sauce thickens then bring to the boil and simmer for 2 to 3 minutes.

3. Stir in the sugar and let cool.

4. Separate the egg and beat the yolk into the sauce mixture.

5. Then whisk the egg white until it is stiff and fold into sauce mixture.

6. Spoon the mixture into a buttered ramekin dish and bake at 400°F, 200°C or Gas Mark 6 for 15 to 20 minutes until golden brown.

7. Remove from the oven and serve at once.

Bread & Butter Pudding

3	Slices	White Bread
1	Cup	Evaporated Milk
1	Medium	Egg
1	Tablespoon	Butter
¼	Cup	Raisins
1	Tablespoon	Mixed Dried Fruit
1	Tablespoon	Sugar

1. Spread the bread with the butter.
2. Cut into quarters and place in a small ovenproof dish.
3. Sprinkle the mixed dried fruit over the bread.
4. Mix together the milk, egg, and sugar.
5. Pour over bread and let soak for a few minutes.
6. Bake in a moderate oven at 350°F, 180°C or Gas Mark 4 for about 35 to 40 minutes.
7. Serve at once.

Baby Pineapple Boats

1	Baby	Pineapple
½	Cup	Cottage Cheese
1	Tablespoon	Chopped Walnuts
1	Pinch	Salt & Pepper

1. Cut the baby pineapple in half lengthways leaving the green top on.

2. Remove the pineapple flesh carefully to leave a boat shape.

3. Chop up the pineapple flesh discarding any core.

4. In a bowl mix together the cheese, salt, pepper, walnuts and the chopped pineapple.

5. Spoon the mixture back into one half of the pineapple skins and chill well in a refrigerator before serving.

6. Remove from the refrigerator and eat at once

Eating Healthfully While Eating Out

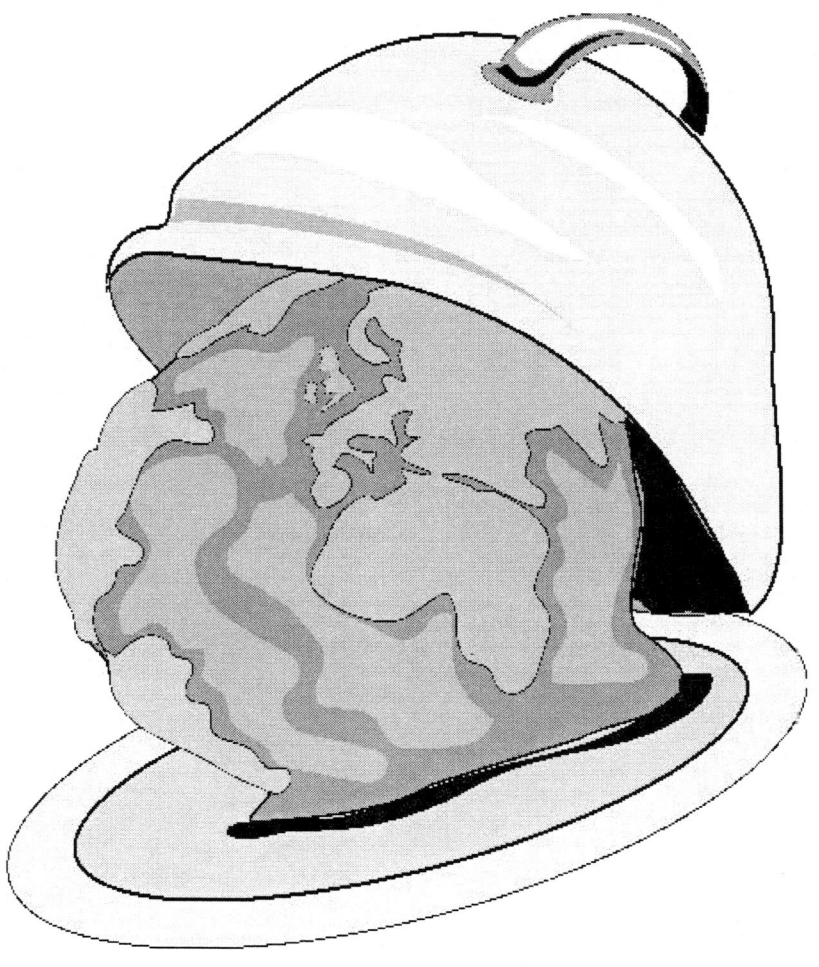

Eating Healthfully While Eating Out

Eating out can present special problems such as those tempting menu choices and portion sizes. Then normally professional kitchens just do not use low fat cooking methods as standard practice. As a rule those less expensive restaurants are more likely to use very generous amounts of fat and high fat cooking techniques as an inexpensive and easy way to add flavour to food. There is the waiting in the bar until your table is ready, so by the time you get to your table your will be ravenous. And then there is the impulse to clean your plate either because the cost of your meal or not to cause offence. But please do take heart there are many ways around all these predicaments. If you eat out frequently for business or pleasure consider becoming a regular at one restaurant this way the staff and kitchen can get to know your taste. This will help so that the kitchen will not be thrown by your special requests.

Chinese

Chinese, eating at a restaurant or as a take-away try to simply eat the way the Chinese do, it is the rice that is the centrepiece of their meal, and diners eat from their rice bowls, not from plates, with the vegetables and meat being selected from the serving dishes, and added to the bowl, and eaten with the rice. Try using chopsticks it can be fun and if you just cannot pass up on an especially fatty dish, be sure to balance it with very lean ones.

Try to select from these for a starter:
- Bean curd broth soup
- Chicken and sweetcorn soup
- Hot and sour soup
- Chinese prawn cocktail
- Sesame 2 prawn on toast 2 pieces

Try to select from these for a main course:
- Steamed prawns with ginger and spring onions
- Prawn chop suey
- Beef with green pepper or mushroom
- Mixed vegetable chop suey
- Plain soft noodle
- Boiled rice
- Bean curd unless fried
- Fish, shrimp, and scallops

Sandwich Meals

You cannot only find good health sandwiches at delicatessens but in most high street stores. You will be confronted with wide range of sandwiches to meat all tastes. So what to buy if it is to your taste go for brown sliced bread, or a bagel and with any of these fillings.

In the shapers, healthy choice or eating range etc,
- Bacon, lettuce
- Tuna, and cucumber
- Tuna, tomato and spring onion
- Tuna and salad
- Brie and grapes
- Chicken salad
- Chicken, tikka
- Roast or smoked turkey
- Prawn, apple and celery
- Prawn, cocktail
- Prawn, mayonnaise
- Egg salad
- Salmon and cucumber
- Roast pork with apple stuffing
- Roast pork salad
- Roast beef salad
- Soft cheese and pineapple
- Mixed salad
- Houmous, carrot and peppers
- Vegetable tikka
- Vegetarian cheese
- Mushroom, onion, tomato and watercress

Fast Food

I am sure on other diets you would have to swear never to eat another burger, fish, chips, french fries, pie, or shake again, but lets face it a trip to the shopping centre or to buy fuel for your vehicle usually means passing fast food outlets, with their aroma trying to seducing you to stop. So if you just can't pass them by this time what to buy. A good start is to buy a very large diet drink, or a can, as this will fill you up.

Try to select from these:
- Bacon and egg McMuffin
- Egg McMuffin
- Chicken McNuggets 4 or 6
- Vegetable burger
- Regular or kid-size single burger
- Regular french fries
- Baked potato with butter
- Baked potato with cottage cheese and chives
- Baked potato with sweetcorn
- Baked potato with bake beans
- Baked potato with tuna
- Chicken for one with coleslaw
- Small portion of chips
- Fishcake
- Scamp in breadcrumbs
- Haddock in batter
- Cod in batter
- Jumbo sausage
- Mushy peas
- Curry sauce
- Pickle egg

Pizza

Pizza is a real plus for dieters as you can add or subtract ingredients to fit your particular tastes. Meat can be chosen from pepperoni, sausage, and bacon to grilled chicken and shrimp. You even can specify the variety of cheese you like so even a traditional pizzeria can be diet friendly if you order selectively. Try to start with a small salad order it with a vinaigrette and please do eat your pizza crust ends as the crust is a good source of low fat, filling carbohydrates.

Try to select from these:
- Ham
- Mushrooms
- Pepperonata
- Grilled chicken
- Strongly flavoured cheeses (you will use less)
- Shrimp
- Tuna
- Vegetable toppings, especially broccoli and spinach

Try not to select from these:
- Bacon
- Extra cheese
- Extra olive oil
- Meatballs
- Olives
- Pepperoni sausage
- Eggs
- Dough balls

French

French cuisine pitfall to people trying to lose weight is the amount of butter and cream in the sauces, its rich salad dressings, and desserts. Even an order of lean meats and fishes will have that wonderful classic butter enhanced sauces. I think you will be very hard pressed to find diet friendly French cuisine. So what to order try to start with a green salad but easy on the dressing or a clear soup

Try to select from these:
Bouillabaisse, (a highly seasoned fish stew made with at least two kinds of fish)
Moules mariniers
Steak au poivre
Steak tartare
Porc aux pruneaux
Food that is (Au vapour) steamed
Food that is (En brochette) skewered and broiled
Food that is (Grillé) grilled
With sour cream yoghurt (Crème fraîche)

Try not to select from these:
In cream sauce (A la crème)
In a pastry crust (En croûte)
With ice cream (A la mode)
Baked with cheese and cream (Au gratin or gratinée)
Remoulade (a mayonnaise-based sauce)

Indian

Many styles of Indian cooking are vegetarian, however it does use lots of a clarified butter called ghee in cooking. You have roasting in a clay oven called a tandoor this is a good low fat cooking method, but other dishes are often stewed and fried. You will be temped by the many Indian breads ranging from chapati to high fat, to deep-fried poori. Indian cuisine uses carbohydrates such as basmati rice and lentils, as its foundation and vegetables are a part of almost every dish, and the sauces are enriched with yoghurt, not cream. So what to choose try to look for these when ordering.

Try to select from these:
- Chicken tandoori or chicken tikka
- King prawn curry
- Vegetable biryani
- Vegetable balti
- Vegetable curry
- Dahl (lentils)
- Tandoori (bake in an clay oven)
- Masala (curry)
- Matta (peas)
- Paneer (a fresh milk cheese)
- Pullao or pilau (rice)
- Raita (a yoghurt and cucumber condiment)

Try not to select from these:
- Korma (cream sauce)
- Ghee (clarified butter)
- Molee (coconut)
- Poori (a deep-fried bread)
- Samosas (fried turnover appetizers)

Italian

In most Italian restaurants portions are generous, and those antipasto (Italian hors d'oeuvres) then the cheese, marinated vegetables, salami, and garlic breads

Try to select from these:
- Bean and pasta soup
- Minestrone
- Calamari (squid)
- Pepperoni ripieni (stuffed peppers)
- Spaghetti vongole (clams)
- Light red sauce
- Marinara sauce
- Pasta (other than those stuffed with cheese)
- Piccata (lemon-wine sauce)
- White or red clam sauce (but ask the wait staff; some clam sauces are made with cream)
- Wine sauce

Try not to select from these:
- Alfredo
- Alla panna (with cream)
- Butter
- Carbonara (butter, eggs, bacon, and sometimes cream sauce)
- Fried aubergine eggplant or zucchini
- Frito misto (fried mixed vegetables or seafood)
- Olive oil
- Parmigiana (baked in sauce with cheese)
- Prosciutto
- Salami

Japanese

Japanese food can be a dieters dream as Japanese can be one of the healthiest cuisines, with only a very few fattening dishes. The main cooking techniques are grilling, steaming, braising or simmering. The portions are small with rice and noodles being the foundation.

Try to select from these:
- Clear broth
- Mushimono (steamed)
- Nabemono (a one-pot dish)
- Nimono (simmered)
- Sashimi
- Sushi
- Udon (noodles)
- Yaki (broiled)
- Yakimono (grilled)

Try not to select from these:
- Agemono (deep fried)
- Katsu (fried pork cutlet)
- Sukiyaki (a one-dish meal made with fatty beef)
- Tempura (batter-fried)

Mexican

Mexican cuisine places minimum importance on meat protein which is fine but as most Mexican food is fried or cooked in lots and lots of fat a flour tortilla is fine on its own, but when it is roll around a filling and deep fried you have a caloric disaster. Ask for cheese toppings to be omitted, or ask if low-fat sour cream and cheese are available. Try to use salsa instead of salad dressing, guacamole, or sour cream on entrees.

Try to select from these:
- Black bean soup
- Ceviche
- Chili
- Enchiladas
- Burritos
- Soft tacos
- Fajitas
- Gazpacho
- Mexican salad

Try not to select from these:
- Chimichangas
- Extra Cheese
- Refried beans
- Sour cream
- Tortilla shells

Thai

Like many Asian cuisines Thai food has rice and noodles, as their staple dishes with all their food being either stir-fried, steamed, braised, or marinated one exception being Thai curry, which is made with coconut milk.

Try to select from these:
- Tom Yum Goong
- Khao Soy (Chiang Mai Noodles)
- Pad See You (Thai Soy Sauce Noodles)
- Pad Thai
- Goong Gah Tiem (Garlic Shrimp)
- Sâté (skewered and grilled meats)
- Basil sauce
- Bean thread noodles
- Fish sauce
- Lime sauce
- Sizzling
- Thai salad

Airline Food

You can order a special meal for a flight as long as you give the airline 24 hours notice. Each airline will have a selection of special menus to accommodate your religious or medical dietary restrictions, or the special needs you have for an infant or child.

You should be able select from these:
- Asian vegetarian meal
- Infant or baby's meal
- Bland/soft meal
- Child's meal
- Diabetic meal
- Fruit platter meal
- Gluten-free meal
- Hindu meal
- Kosher meal
- Low-calorie meal
- Low-cholesterol/low-fat meal
- Low-sodium meal
- Muslim meal
- Oriental meal
- Vegetarian meal (non-dairy)
- Vegetarian meal (lacto-ovo)
- Strict Vegetarian
- Vegan
- Non-lactose meal
- Fruit Plate
- Seafood

Exercise

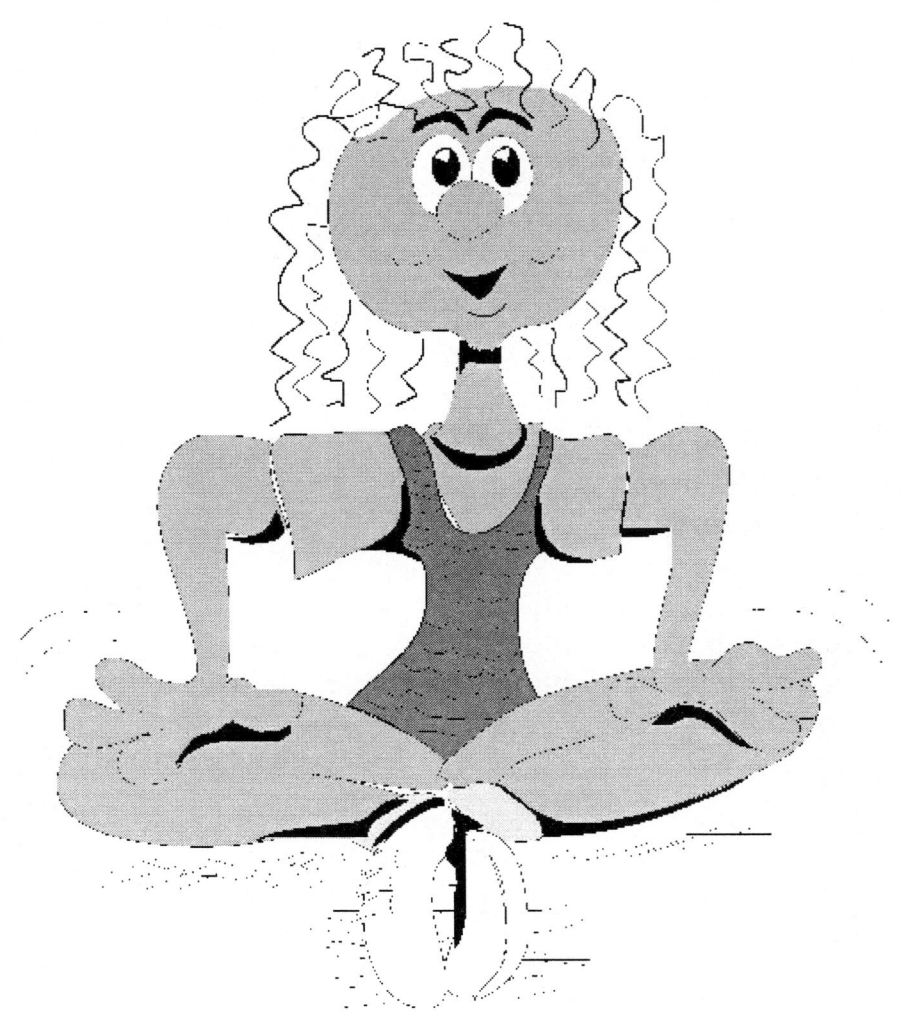

Exercise

You already should know that exercise is important; and that it can reduce your risk of medical problems, the psychological benefits of exercise, and how it can improving your looks. When you start an exercise plan it is always helpful to remind yourself just why you are do this. Even if you are at this time a committed exerciser, you probably will still have moments when you say I am just too tired or too busy, or the dog ate your shoes. Any time you experience one of these moments just remember why and who you are doing this for.

- Regular exercise makes you less tense and better able to cope with what life thoughts at you, as you will experience less stress.
- Weight training prevents your muscles from wasting away as you slim down, and aerobic exercise is the most efficient way to burn calories.
- You are more likely to keep the weight off, as more than 95 percent of those whom work out regularly will keep the pounds off.
- You are less likely to get diabetes as staying fit can drastically reduces your chances of developing non-insulin dependent diabetes by lowering blood sugar and blood fat levels. And if you do have diabetes, exercise with the permission of a doctor can help control the symptoms.
- You discover abilities you never knew you had
- You can eat more without gaining weight when you burn extra calories a week on your fitness plan
- You can enjoy life more being just a bit fitter
- Moderate daily exercise, such as an hour long walk or a half hour jog, may reduce your colon cancer risk by as much as 46 percent.

Both men and women start losing bone mass between the ages of 30 and 40 but by lifting weights can not only halt the decline but in some cases can reverse it, drastically reducing your risk for osteoporosis.

- Walking and running can also help keep your bones strong.
- You will sleep more soundly by exercising regularly you boost the amount of time spent in slow-wave sleep, the phase of sleep believed to be the most restorative.
- You are less likely to catch a cold because even moderate exercise strengthens your immune system.
- People who walk regularly report cold symptoms on fewer than half the days that couch potatoes report symptoms.
- You're more likely to live a long life.
- Even fat men who were fit had a lower death rate than those who were lean but unfit.
- People who complain that they do not have enough energy to exercise fail to realize that working out gives you energy.
- You lessen the symptoms of PMS exercise may reduce the bloating, lower back pain, headaches, and anxiety that often accompany premenstrual syndrome.
- Regular exercisers may be less likely to experience PMS at all.
- In one study, middle-aged women who lifted weights for a year became 27 percent more active in daily life than before.
- You have more energy.
- You can ease the symptoms of menopause, as highly active women are significantly less likely to experience hot flushes than their counterparts it has been found that an aerobic workout is a great mood boost.
- You can expand your social horizons even if you are not on the hunt for a spouse, getting into a new fitness activity is a great way to widen your social circle.

Research suggests that physically active women are less prone to breast cancer than women who don't work out.

- You improve your memory. In a six-month study of previously sedentary men and women ages 60 to 75, those who walked three times a week scored 25 percent better on memory and judgment tasks.

- You lower your risk of coronary heart disease; people who do not exercise are as likely to develop heart disease as those people who smoke.

- You improve your balance. In just three months, 80-year-olds who performed balance exercises -- like walking a straight line and standing on one foot -- gained the level of body control typical of people three to ten years younger. With improved balance, you have a zippier walking gait as you age, and less shuffling means fewer falls and fractures.

- You're less likely to have a stroke. Burning more than 1,000 calories per week through exercise (say, walking four hours a week) is associated with decreased stroke risk. Burning between 2,000 and 3,000 calories per week may lower your risk even more

- Not only will a single workout make you feel better, but also regular exercisers enjoy long-lasting psychological benefits.

- You can cope better with shift work as exercise can help temper the health problems, including sleep disorders, common to people who work shifts.

- You have fewer tension headaches it has been found that people with chronic tension headaches feel better when they work out.

- Regular aerobic exercise appears to lower levels of LDL cholesterol.

- Some research suggests that exercise may also raise levels of HDL, the good cholesterol.

You lower your resting heart rate when you work out on a regular basis; your heart beats fewer times per minute to pump the same amount of blood.

- You enjoy retirement more as fit seniors have more activity choices, from golf to gardening to world travel.
- You're less likely to get a stress fracture.
- You will gain confidence that spills over to the rest of your life as the sense of accomplishment that comes from being able fit.
- You set a good example for your kids.
- You can be a great role model by exercising regularly.
- You are more likely to stop smoking people who exercise vigorously while trying to kick the habit are twice as likely to stay away from cigarettes as ex-smokers who do not work out.
- You can relieve arthritic pain not only can arthritis patients safely participate in exercise programs, but they often are rewarded for their efforts with pain relief and increased mobility.
- So you can keep up with your grandchildren.
- Your pet will get fit, too as you will be able to take you're dog for longer and more frequent walks, and he will live a longer, healthier life.

The Exercise Plan

We can be find creative ways to incorporate movement into almost everything we do no matter where or who we are here are some suggestions:

- Loose the TV remote.

- Walk up the stairs instead of the lift.

- During breaks at work, walk around the building.

- Whenever you are walking try to focus on long strides and a quicker than normal pace.

- Unless it is urgent, always opt for the bathroom that is furthest from you, same for answering the telephone.

- When cleaning house, exaggerate your movements.

- Work in the garden.

- If you have children, or grandchildren, spend some quality time playing with them.

- Few things can jump-start your heart as quickly as trying to keep up with a child play catch, jump rope, push them on the swing.

Proper Clothing for Specific Activity

Proper clothing is just as important as all the other requirements for effective exercise.

- Running shoes provide the needed heel cushioning but lack in the side-to-side lateral support for required for aerobics so you should buy aerobic shoes.
- It is important to wear clothing that allows the skin to breathe as the body utilizes sweating to regulate temperature so clothes that restrict the cooling of the skin are not recommended.
- It is important to wear clothing that allows the body to ventilate because if evaporation does not occur, the wet clothing will continue to help radiate body heat.
- This can lead to loss of excess body heat after exercise when heat retention is important.
- Cotton soaks up sweat readily, but stays wet. Wool, however, continues to provide body warmth even when wet but nylon does not allow water to permeate through.
- Obviously, layers are important in cold weather environments. Layers allow you to remove and replace outer garments as the need arises.
- Hats are equally important in cold weather since a considerable amount of body heat can be lost through the head.
- In warm weather, wear loose clothing that allows sweat evaporation.

Basic Step Moves

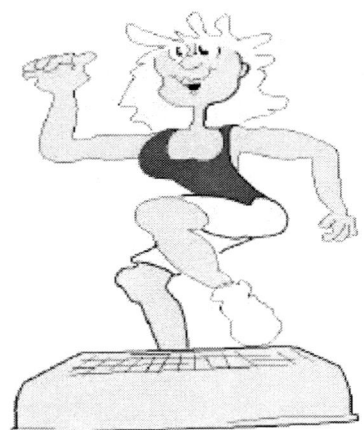

- General Technique
  - Step up with whole foot flat on the board.
  - Step off board to floor with toe to heel.
  - Slight lean forward at the waist.
  - Heels stay off floor during lunges.

Basic Left (Reverse for Basic Right)

Basic left is one of the simplest and most basic of all step moves

- Start Position
  - Centred in front of the bench.

- Description
  - Step up on the bench with the left foot
  - Step up on the bench with the right foot
  - Step down left foot, then down right foot.

- Count Breakdown:
  1. Step up on bench with left foot
  2. Step up on bench with right foot
  3. Step down backwards to the floor with left foot
  4. Step down backwards to the floor with right foot

V-Step

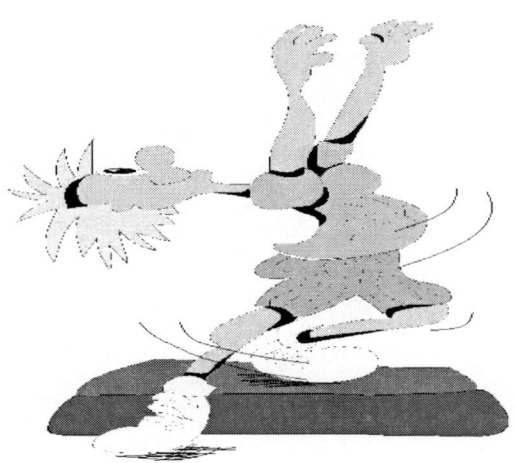

Feet together on the floor, and spread apart while on the bench

- Start Position
    - o Centered in front of the bench.

- Description
    - o Like a basic but step wide on the bench.

- Count Breakdown:
    1. Step up on bench with leading foot as wide as possible
    2. Step up on bench with the other foot as wide as possible
    3. Step down backwards to the floor with lead foot
    4. Step down backwards to the floor with left foot

A-Step

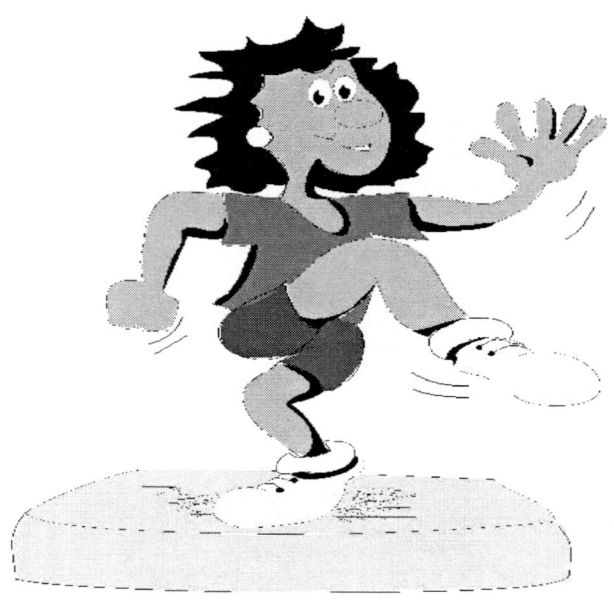

Start and end with feet together on opposite ends of the bench.

- Start Position
    - In front of the bench, but off to one side.

- Description
    - This is a modified basic step in the shape of a letter A

- Count Breakdown:
    1. Step up with leading foot at the center of the bench
    2. Step up with the other foot next to the lead foot
    3. Step down backwards to the floor with lead foot
    4. Step down backwards to the floor with left foot

Turn Step

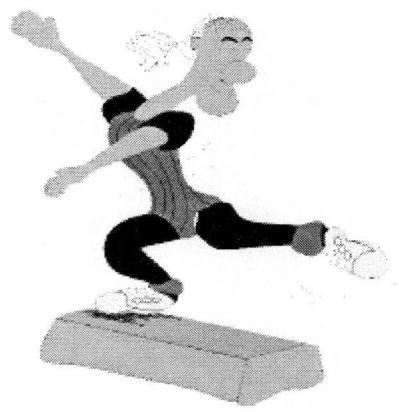

- <u>Start Position</u>
  - In front of the bench, but off to one side.

- <u>Description</u>
  - Start on side of bench and do a modified basic while turning.

- <u>Count Breakdown:</u>
  1. Step up on the bench with the left foot
  2. Step up on the bench with the right foot while turning to the left
  3. Step off the bench with left foot, turn to the left slightly
  4. Bring the right foot down on the floor next to your left
  5. Step up on the bench with the right foot
  6. Step up on the bench with the left foot while turning to the right
  7. Step off the bench with the right foot, turn to the right slightly
  8. Bring the left foot down on the floor next to the right

Z-Step

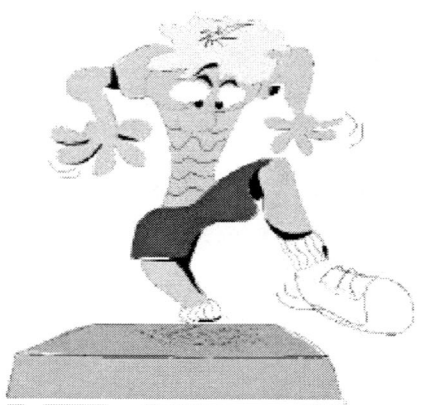

When left foot leads, counts 3-8 for the letter Z

- <u>Start Position</u>
  - Centred in front of the bench.

- <u>Description</u>
  - Step across the bench, off diagonally, and across the floor to form the letter Z.

- <u>Count Breakdown:</u>
  1. Step onto left side of bench with left foot
  2. Step up with right foot next to the left (feet are together on the left side of the bench)
  3. Step to the right side of the bench with right foot
  4. Step to the right side of bench with left foot (feet are together on the right side of the bench)
  5. Step back diagonally to the ground with left foot (left foot is now in front of the bench on the far left side)
  6. Step back diagonally to the ground with the right foot (feet are together on the left and on the floor)
  7. Step on the floor to the right with right foot
  8. Step on the floor to the right with left foot (feet are together on the left and on the floor)

X-Step

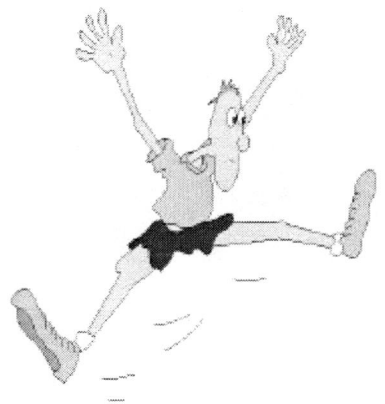

- Start Position
    - Straddling the bench.

- Description
    - Start from a straddle position at one end of the bench.

- Count Breakdown:
    1. Step up to centre of bench with right foot
    2. Step up to centre of bench with left foot
    3. Step down and forward with right foot to the floor on the right side of the bench
    4. Step down and forward with left foot to the floor on the left side of the bench
    5. Step up and backward to the centre of the bench with right foot
    6. Step up and backward to the centre of the bench with left foot
    7. Step down and backward with right foot to the floor on the right side of the bench
    8. Step down and backward with left foot to the floor on the left side of the bench

Kickbox Aerobics

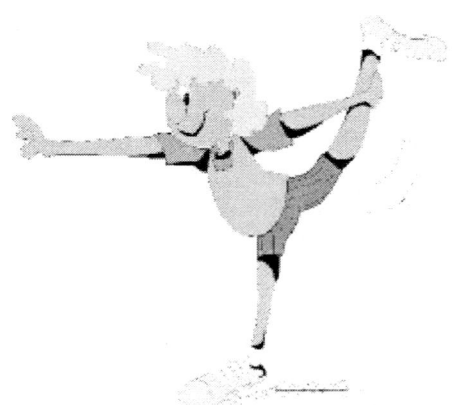

- <u>Warm Up</u>
    - Begin with wide stance deep breaths to oxygenate the blood.
    - March in place, side step, grapevine.
    - Include wide stance toe tapping with reach out and up.
    - Extend reach across the centreline of the body.
    - Transition from reaching up and out to jabs to the front.
    - Include hook punches.

- <u>General Technique</u>
    - Chin is tucked in and down.
    - Don't aim for the target, aim behind the target.
    - Always look in the direction of the punch or kick before executing.
    - Extend shoulder into the punch.
    - Keep abdominal tight to improve muscle tone and balance.
    - Keep fists in front of face when not punching. (Defence Position)

- <u>Boxer's Stance Technique</u>
    - Stay light on the feet to keep impact to a minimum.
    - Maintain a rocking back and forth motion.

- Keep heels lightly touching the floor.
- Keep weight on the ball of the foot.
- Keep fists in front of face when not punching. (Defence Position)
- Discontinue is joint pain or discomfort is experienced.
- Stay on Boxer's Stance for no more than 5 minutes at a time.
- Provide lower impact exercise for at least 5 minutes in between.

- Safety
  - Limit Kickboxing Aerobics tempo range from 120 - 125 bpm.
  - Limit warm-up tempo range from 120 - 134 bpm.
  - Limit cool-down music tempo range from 118 - 122 bpm.
  - Avoid moves that require back kicks in a crowded class.
  - Lock knees to provide shock absorption and reduce back strain.
  - Limit power moves (propulsion) to 1-minute intervals.
  - Limit repeater moves to five repeaters at time.
  - The more advanced students can use lightweights.
  - Instructor should avoid using weights.
  - Avoid pivoting moves on a loaded knee.
  - Unlike Step multiple moves are permitted.(i.e., legs and arms)
  - Always provide low impact alternatives to high impact moves.
  - Continue breathing, never hold the breath.
  - Instruct class to work at their own pace, not the instructor's.

Discontinue Kickbox Aerobics if:
- Legs become fatigued and uncoordinated.
- Any pain becomes evident especially joint pain.
- Shin area pain or discomfort.
- Dizziness occurs.
- Rapid heart rate.

Using and Buying Aerobic Machines

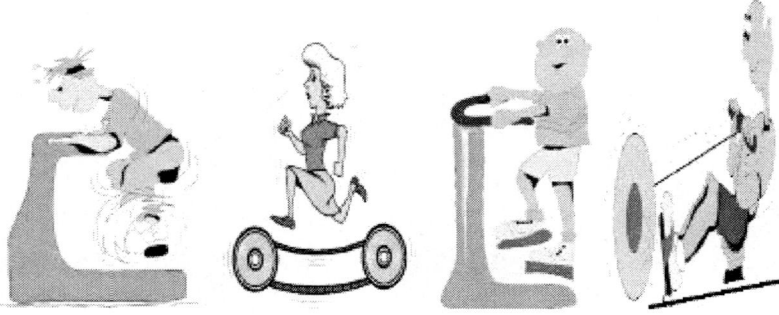

Home aerobic equipment has become very imagined in their designs some having a computer display worthy of a NASA mission. You now can be informed about how far you walked, cycled, steps climbed. You need to identify your fitness needs and the available space for it to live.

- The equipment should suit your interests and fitness level and any disability you may have.

- You need to chosen an activity that you find enjoyable and yet challenging enough so that you are able to progress to higher levels.

- You should be able to increase the resistance, incline or duration of a given piece of equipment.

- If the goal is an aerobic workout, then the equipment's resistance should be low enough to maintain at least 20 minutes of smooth continuous motion. If the goal is muscle strengthening, then considerably more resistance is required. For this reason, it's difficult to obtain muscle strengthening benefits and aerobic benefits from the same piece of equipment. In most cases, machines that claim to do both (riders for example) are inadequate for strengthening beyond the initial level of sedentary beginners.

- Determine your budget but the rule here is that you only get what you pay for.

You need to keep in mind that high quality equipment that works reliably after several years of heavy use cannot be manufactured cheaply.

- In some cases in fact the price range on a particular piece of equipment can vary wildly so it is important to do your homework and find out what the best price is.

- By the same token, if a piece of equipment is priced significantly higher than comparably models, you need to ask why, such as does it work better than lower priced models? Does it offer better and more features

- Keep in mind that it's possible to purchase used exercise equipment. If you go this route, you may be able to buy more equipment, or higher quality commercial equipment, and still stay within your budget.

- Determine how much space there is available taking into consideration the room usage, safety, traffic flow, aesthetics, desired equipment, and future expansion possibilities.

- Plan for at least as much open space as equipment space.

- Use the following guidelines to determine how much room you'll need:

  - Treadmills about 30 square feet
  - Bikes about 10 square feet
  - Single Station Gym about 35 square feet
  - Multi Station Gym about 50-200 square feet
  - Rowing Machines about 20 square feet
  - Free Weights about 20-50 square feet
  - Stair Climbers about 10-20 square feet
  - Ski Machines about 25 square feet

- The equipment should be adjustable, comfortable, easy to learn, and able to fit users of various sizes.

- Parts should be easily removed and replaced.

The device should be space-efficient, and the components should be the highest quality in the price range.

- Think about the advertising claims. They should be backed up by solid research. Look for reviews by objective consumer publications.

- Moving parts should mesh well. Welds should be clean and smooth and the frame should be thick and sturdy.

- Check out the safety features. There shouldn't be any design flaws or weaknesses that increase the risk of injury.

- Look for features that enhance safety. For example, range-of-motion limiters on strength machines; weight-stack guards or any guards that protect moving parts; safety switches on treadmills.

- Using this quick checklist as a side-by side comparison tool:
  - Price
  - Safety
  - Effectiveness
  - Comfort and enjoy ability
  - Space efficiency
  - Adjustability
  - Durable design
  - Quiet operation
  - A guide on how to use it
  - Reputable manufacturer
  - Written warranty
  - Service plan and parts availability

Maintenance Plan

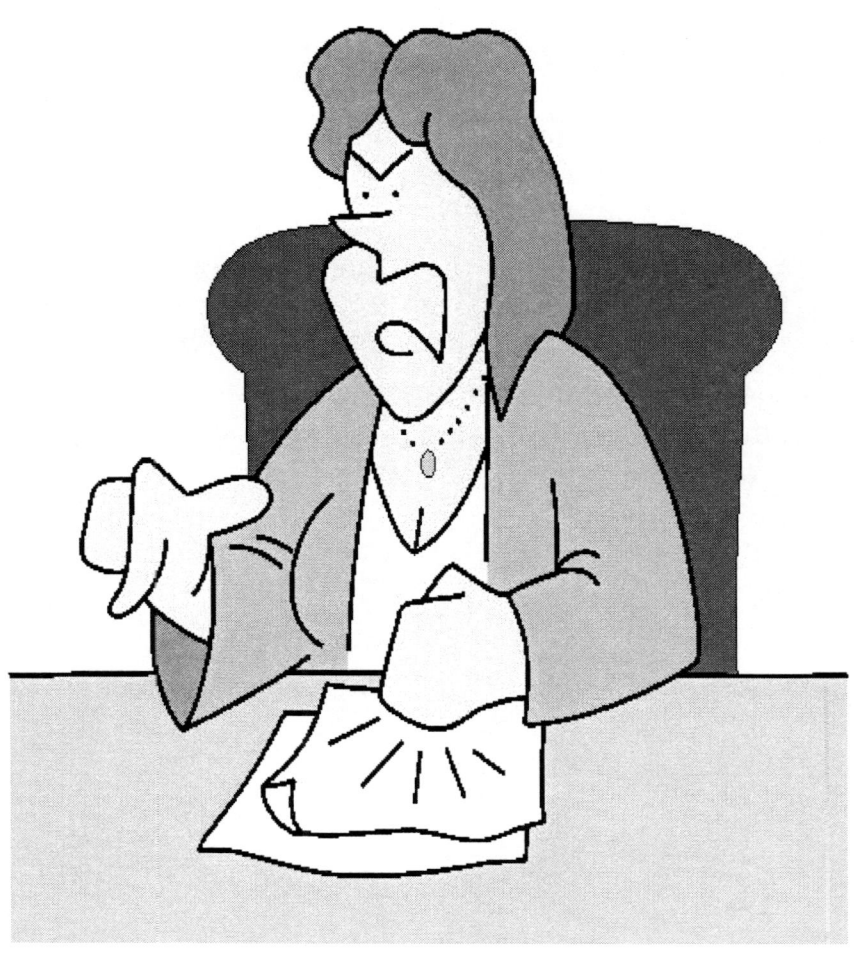

Diets Maintenance Plan

Weight your self once a week only at the same time of day wearing the same type of clothing.

On reaching your desired weight just add a small snack daily for the next four weeks monitoring your weight weekly?

If your weight starts to go up more them a few pounds check what you are eating and drop back for a week only then move back to adding a small snack daily for the next four weeks.

After your weight remaining constant for four weeks move back on to adding a light meal daily for the next eight weeks again monitoring your weight weekly?

If your weight starts to go up more than a few pounds check what you are eating and drop back for a week only then move back to adding a light meal daily for the next eight weeks.

Now by add a little more each week to what you have been eating on the Diet Plan and again monitoring your weight weekly? You should stay at your new weight.

Congratulations I knew we could do it together.

Web Site Details and Links

Cooking tips are available from the Forest of Dean web site at:
http://www.recipes4one.co.uk/cooktips.htm

Additional recipes are available for free from:
http://www.recipes4one.co.uk /recipes.htm

We run an online diet club were you are able to get help and talk to other users of the diet plans:
http://clubs.yahoo.com/clubs/forestofdeandietplan

We offer for your guidance an online:

BMI Calculator:
http:// www.recipes4one.co.uk /bmi.htm

Body Calculator:
http:// www.recipes4one.co.uk /bodyfat.htm

Calories Burner Calculator:
http:// www.recipes4one.co.uk /burner.htm

For further details of the "FOD" Diet Plans send an email to:
dietinfo@recipes4one.co.uk

Index